Contents

Life in a Hospice
Reflections on caring for the dying

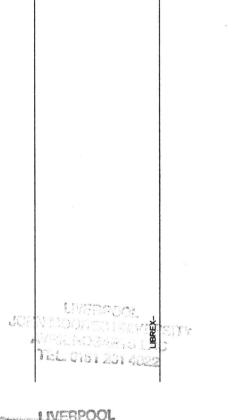

Radcliffe Publishing
Oxford • New York

Radcliffe Publishing Ltd
18 Marcham Road
Abingdon
Oxon OX14 1AA
United Kingdom

www.radcliffe-oxford.com
Electronic catalogue and worldwide online ordering facility.

British Library Cataloguing in Publication Data

A catalogue record for this book is available from the British Library.

ISBN-13: 978 1 84619 243 2

Typeset by Phoenix Photosetting, Chatham, Kent
Printed and bound by TJI Digital, Padstow, Cornwall

Foreword

This is a book about the care provided by hospices. I am a passionate supporter of the hospice movement. I first heard about hospices when I was in America. I was having dinner at the British Embassy in the late 1960s and an American woman was so enthusiastic that it awakened my interest – and now, of course, it has become a worldwide movement.

My mother, a very religious woman, said death is God's last and greatest gift to the living. Like everybody, I've had many experiences of death. When I was 10, my mother had a stillborn baby who she grieved over for years. That made a huge impression on me. When my father died, I sat next to him in the hospital. I missed my mother's death by an hour, although I spoke to her that morning on the telephone. And my wife Caroline died of cancer seven years ago. That was a tremendously moving experience. The pain and the grief are not something you can talk about easily. Of course, you cannot fill the gap that is left, but you can decorate the gap with your happy memories.

The hospice movement says to the dying 'abide with us', as spelled out in the beautiful hymn 'Abide with me':

> 'Abide with me, fast falls the eventide,
> The darkness deepens, Lord with me abide.
> When other helpers fail and comforts flee
> Help of the helpless, abide with me.'

Hospices provide palliative care, which tells you to think about the person, rather than the disease. It is important to address people's real problems. And if you can make it possible to die without worrying, that is so much better than dying with a lot of pain. This book is full of examples of such care and attention. Indeed, the idea of palliative care has a significance beyond the hospice movement – I think I have been in palliative politics all my life.

The more I think about the hospice movement, the more I feel the issue is not *dying* well, but *living* well until you die. The hospice movement loves the living right up to the point when they die. I was in Paddington station recently and there was a group of young people with cardboard signs offering 'free hugs'. A girl of 17 gave me a hug. And an old lady with white hair was warmly hugged by a boy of about 16. The free hug movement seems to me to be what hospices are about – it's love.

Sogyal Rinpoche, a Tibetan Buddhist, has said:

'When we finally know we are dying, and all other sentient beings are dying with us, we start to have a burning, almost heartbreaking sense of the fragility and preciousness of each moment and each being. And from this can grow a deep, clear, limitless compassion for all beings.'

That is what the hospice movement is about. That is what this important book is about. I recommend it strongly.

Tony Benn
July 2007

Preface

This book has had a very long gestation period. Nearly 20 years ago, I met a man who had worked as an AIDS nurse – and who subsequently died from the disease – and he talked a lot to me about the emotional difficulties of nursing the dying. I was immediately drawn to wondering how it affected people to spend their day-to-day lives working with dying people. Later, I worked briefly in a hospice as a volunteer, and experienced at first hand some of the rewards of such work and some of the complexities of that environment. It occurred to me that it would make an interesting book, but that is as far as I got.

In fact, the hurdles involved in writing a book of this kind are considerable. I knew that I would need to get the permission of one or two hospices, to find interviewers willing to take on the task, to interest a publisher sufficiently to make the project worth embarking on, to undergo the cumbersome process of obtaining 'ethical approval' required (at that time) for almost any research connected to the NHS and, finally, to gain funding to cover my expenses. I did what any sensible person would do and put my intellectual energies to easier tasks.

But eventually, the lure of this book proved too strong. Almost by accident, I obtained the permission of one hospice – and then sought out and found another. I put together a proposal and found, to my delight, that two publishers were keen to publish the proposed manuscript. Interviewers were fairly easy to find, as I work with several who were likely to find this work interesting. It took roughly six months to obtain the necessary ethical approval. And, despite considerable efforts, I never did get any external funding.

I undertook this project because I thought it would be fascinating. What makes people want to work in a hospice day after day? What is it like to help patients and their families at this vulnerable time? What aspects of such work are most difficult and what enables people to cope? And what is the impact on their lives at home? I felt if such questions were intriguing to myself, they might also be intriguing to other lay people. And, of course, those already working in palliative care – or others with an interest in doing so – might welcome the opportunity to reflect on this work. It is my hope that all readers will find something of interest in this book.

For readers new to the subject, it may be useful to provide some very brief information. There are roughly 250 hospices in the UK, most of which are for adults but a small number are solely for children. These are run by a variety of organisations, primarily local charities. The following description of hospice care is courtesy of Help the Hospices, the national charity supporting hospices, and can be found on the Hospice Information website (www.hospiceinformation.info/whatishospice):

Hospice care is one of the UK's outstanding success stories. From the opening of the first modern hospice, St Christopher's, in south London in 1967, it has grown into a worldwide movement that has radically changed the way we approach death and dying. It is regarded by some as one of the greatest social innovations of the last hundred years.

The driving force behind hospice, or palliative, care is the desire to transform the experience of dying. Still in the 21st century in the UK people die in avoidable pain and distress. In hospices, multi-disciplinary teams strive to offer freedom from pain, dignity, peace and calm at the end of life.

Underpinning this care is a philosophy that takes as its starting point the affirmation of death as a natural part of life. Built on that bedrock are the values of respect, choice, empowerment, holistic care and compassion. Hospices care for the whole person, aiming to meet all needs – physical, emotional, social and spiritual. They care for the person who is dying and for those who love them, at home, in day care and in the hospice. Nearly half of all people admitted to a hospice return home again. The average length of stay is just 13 days. All care is free of charge.

Within hospices you will find a range of services – pain control, symptom relief, skilled nursing care, counselling, complementary therapies, spiritual care, art, music, physiotherapy, reminiscence, beauty treatments and bereavement support.

Staff and volunteers work in multi-professional teams to provide care based on individual need and personal choice.

It will be seen that this book illustrates these values time and again.

Many a novel starts with the disclaimer 'the characters and events in this novel are fictitious – any similarity to real persons, dead or alive, is wholly coincidental' or words to that effect. In this book, the complete opposite is the case. The people in this book are all very real – actual nurses, doctors, managers and others who have chosen to work in a hospice. The stories they tell concern real events and real patients they have known. The feelings they recount are genuine and personal. All agreed to take part in an interview about their work and its impact on their lives. And all agreed, after the interview, to the publication of the passages shown.

But interviews, if undertaken with some sensitivity, can serve almost as a confessional. They provide an opportunity for people to reflect on their day-to-day lives and speak openly about thoughts or feelings that they might not otherwise make public. This certainly happened in this case. As a result, considerable effort has been taken to anonymise those speaking here. All names have been changed, as well as minor details, to avoid identification. Moreover, two different systems for identifying them have been employed. When people describe their work (Chapters 1–5), their professional title is used, as it is helpful for the reader to know the perspective of the speaker. When they explore more personal matters (Chapters 6–12), however, a pseudonym has been employed. There are a few exceptions, for instance where it is obvious that it is a doctor or chaplain who is talking. This may, at times, appear awkward, but it is preferable to exposing the inner thoughts of people who gave their time freely for this endeavour. They need to be protected from the curious eyes not only of the reading public but also of their colleagues.

So, who did we interview for this book and how were they chosen? I explained to the heads of both hospices the rough nature of the posts we would want to cover and, in one case, staff were invited to volunteer and, in the other, senior staff made suggestions about who should be involved. All were fully informed about what would be required of them and all gave permission for publication, as noted above. All interviews were taped and fully transcribed, which ensured that their actual words made it to the printed page.

In total, we interviewed 31 people. This included the heads of both hospices, twelve nurses covering a range of grades and two healthcare assistants. In addition, we interviewed three chaplains, two hospice doctors, a consultant, a social worker and a variety of therapists, including two counsellors, an occupational therapist and a complementary therapist. There were also people with other very specific jobs, such as the manager of a day centre, a patient affairs officer, a volunteer coordinator and a chef. Two volunteers were included. Occasionally, these posts overlapped.

The question might be asked whether the hospices selected could reasonably be deemed to be 'representative' of all other hospices – and the simple answer is one cannot know. I would make no such claim. The hospices themselves differed in some ways from each other and are likely to differ from others around the country or around the world. Nor can I claim that those interviewed are 'representative' of all hospice staff. They cover a range of positions and views, but in the end, they speak for themselves.

I would like to acknowledge the very great help from my two interviewers, Kit Ward and Paul Vallance, whose sensitivity and skill contributed enormously to the nature of the discussions held. I would also like to thank the London School of Economics and Political Science for providing me a Visiting Fellowship during this time. And, most importantly, I must give my very deep thanks to all the people interviewed who gave their time generously to discuss their work and its impact on their lives.

A brief introduction to the shape of this book may be helpful. It starts with a chapter describing what hospices do – and why the care they provide is different from much hospital care (Chapter 1). The first main section then describes the work undertaken in hospices (Chapters 2–5), including all aspects of patient care but with particular attention to the processes of helping dying people and supporting their relatives after a death. The next section (Chapters 6–8) explores the difficulties entailed in hospice work and the various means employed by staff to cope with them. The third section (Chapters 9–10) addresses the underlying question of why people undertake this work. Finally, the last section offers some reflections on working in a hospice (Chapters 11–12), both in terms of practicalities and, more fundamentally, what has been learned from the experience.

Ann Richardson
July 2007

About the author

Ann Richardson started her career as a junior academic researcher and subsequently worked as a senior researcher at the Policy Studies Institute in the broad area of health and social care. Since the late 1980s, she has made her living as a freelance researcher, writer and editor. In recent years, she has undertaken extensive research for public agencies on patients' experiences of treatment for various diseases, such as cancer, diabetes and coronary heart disease, based on interviews and focus groups. She has also carried out occasional research on doctors' and nurses' views about their work. With regard to palliative care, she has written and edited a number of publications, including helping the team developing national guidance on improving supportive and palliative care in cancer services for the National Institute for Clinical Excellence. She is currently a Visiting Fellow at the London School of Economics and Political Science.

Ann has co-authored two other narrative books: one about people with HIV and AIDS: *Wise Before Their Time: people with AIDS and HIV talk about their lives* (Harper Collins, 1992) and the other about the problems faced by parents with adult sons and daughters with learning disabilities: *Letting Go* (Open University Press, 1989).

CHAPTER 1

Introducing hospices

This is a book about hospices as seen through the eyes of the people who work in them. It explores the nature of their work, some problems they experience and how they cope with them and, most importantly, what makes it all worthwhile. It ends with some reflections on the impact of such work on their own sense of mortality and what they have learned from their experience.

But first it is necessary to address what hospices do and do not do. This chapter introduces the complex nature of hospice work and some ways in which care in hospices may differ from hospital care, touching on a number of themes explored in greater depth in later chapters.

The work of hospices

Perhaps the best place to start is with assumptions about hospices. Most people think that hospices are places where people go to die. This is only partially the case. First, life is unpredictable:

> I met a patient this morning who has been coming to the day centre for two years. I always ask him how he is. I said 'you are looking well' and he said 'I am well – they told me two years ago I had five days, and I have proved them wrong'. I said 'good for you, carry on proving them wrong'. The doctors are brilliant, but many people have come in here and been told they have got months – and a couple of years later they are still going.
>
> *Healthcare assistant 1*

> They don't all come here to die. They do go home. We had a man who came in on a stretcher, very, very poorly – and he walked out. That was great. He had everybody in tears saying goodbye to him. And he hasn't come back.
>
> *Healthcare assistant 2*

Second, hospices do more than care for dying people:

> Nowadays, a hospice is here for terminal care, TLC, pain control, families wanting to go on holidays and leave a patient with us. We are here for all different reasons – we have got a day centre, we have got everything. You could die at home or you can die in the hospice, whatever you choose.
>
> *Nurse 1*

A lot of people think 'this is where I'm going to die' – but it's not necessarily the case. They can be in and out of the hospice having treatment, getting stabilised, or getting their symptoms sorted. Some hospices don't take people till the end stage, but we often know them through the day centre or the community team, so there is a link fairly early on.

Head of hospice 1

There was a young man, only in his early forties, and the social worker had tried desperately to get him in for respite care and pain control. His idea was that you come in and you don't go out. He came for a look round the place and saw that we had Jacuzzis and things and I said 'it's just two weeks – if you want to go after the first day, it's up to you. The point is that you come in for a bit of convalescence, so we can control your pain and then you can go home'. He has now been here for two weeks and, we're on top of his pain.

Discharge nurse 2

And many wrongly think that they are depressing places, full of miserable people:

People say to me 'oh, it must be really, really morbid', but I say no, what you find in a hospice is exactly what you'd find in a family home. There will be laughter and there will be tears, there will be happiness and sadness – those four ingredients make up the hospice, as they do your family home. You are going to hear laughter from one family, then another who are in tears because someone's dying. You don't deny the person laughing the chance to laugh, because that might be their last laugh. The family in tears also acknowledge that, because probably two days before, they were laughing as well. People generally acknowledge that they're all travelling the same journey, but at different times and at a different pace.

Chaplain 2

My mates have asked if it is depressing. I have taken them around the ward to see the patients and they see that it *is* really nice – 'just such a great place'. And that's what the hospice is. People on the outside have this connotation that a hospice is where we shunt people – the lepers and the dying. In fact, these are the happiest people you have ever met – they are getting the best care they can achieve and have counsellors preparing them for the fact that they are going to die.

Chef

If you come in the day centre at about 11.30 in the morning, you can hear the laughter coming out of here. You really wouldn't believe that you were in a place where people were so sick. People are happy to be here. The exercises and the music we play has got a lot to do with it – and they're relieved to be out of their homes, talking to people, and probably just to be alive. We very rarely see tears. I always say we've made laughter a condition of entry. To me, it's been one of the most wonderful experiences of my life to be here.

Volunteer 1

Helping dying people

Of course, hospices do involve death and dying. Every effort is made to enable this to be handled in the way patients want:

> There was a gentleman who wanted to die outside under a tree – and he died under the tree. We took him out in the bed. Fortunately it was in the middle of the night, it was in the early hours, so we could tell when he was close to dying and we just took him out there. One of the nurses said that this was what he wanted and we said 'yes, we'll do that.'
>
> *Senior staff nurse 1*

> A good death is about peace. If we can overcome a person's pain and make them comfortable, they relax. I have witnessed death where people have fought to the last breath – you give them medication after medication and they fight it, because it is almost 'I am not ready to go, I haven't sorted things out yet'. But on the whole, people come in here and it is like they breathe out a sigh of relief and relax. They let us care for them – 99% of the time people die peacefully and not in pain.
>
> *Healthcare assistant 1*

> Recently, we had a woman in her late forties whom we got to know for a while, together with her husband and teenage children. We were planning on getting her home where she wanted to be. And then one morning she wasn't wakening – she deteriorated very quickly and she was dead by lunchtime. But she was very peaceful. Through her expression, you could see she wasn't in pain, she wasn't distressed. She had always said 'well, if I die here, that won't be a problem, because I know you all, so it's not as though I'm with strangers'.
>
> *Senior staff nurse 2*

Great emphasis is placed on getting the most out of their remaining time:

> Palliative care is about knowing that there is nothing else that anybody can do, in the sense of making you better, but it is about making life liveable and enjoyable. Even if you can't talk and even if you can't function physically, it is about making the most of every day – it extends beyond the physical. It goes right through to the family, it is about relationships, it is about living every day to the very last to the best quality.
>
> *Discharge nurse 1*

We may know that within a few days or weeks they're going to die, but until that time, their symptoms are controlled, they feel they're treated with dignity, their pain is taken care of. And their spiritual and psychological issues are addressed – we've even been able to bring estranged families together. We see every patient every day, find out what the problems are, see what they did yesterday, what can we make better today. It's not just the dying – they're *living* before they die.

Doctor 2

Indeed, hospices do not have a death every day:

Sometimes there could be a few deaths over the period of a week, or it could be a couple of weeks before somebody dies. I would be dealing with somebody dying at least once a month, if not more often.

Senior staff nurse 3

There tend to be a few deaths per week. There are a lot of superstitions in nursing, like deaths always go in threes – it's surprising, but they do. You'll have one going, two going and we'll say there has to be a third – and it's not always the most obvious one.

Nurse 2

I worked Friday, Saturday, Sunday nights – and we had one death Friday night. I left here Monday morning at 8 o'clock and I came back Wednesday and there had been five. So you can go a week and then have lots. There's no particular amount – it goes in fits and starts.

Healthcare assistant 2

Activities and therapies
Hospices also provide all kinds of activities in day centres, where people can meet and chat to others in a similar situation:

There are lunches on certain days for people who come here for day care. We supply a three-course lunch. On one day a week, we have a buffet – it started with 30 to 40 people and it's now up to 80 to 100. People come and sit and share experiences. They are all people with some sort of illness, but who are not at the hospice stage now. I go down and have a chat with them, talking about their weekend and about mine. It's like a small friendship.

Chef

I wanted to reach out into the community to get people in, in a very non-threatening way, because people thought this was a black hole that you got swallowed up in. So we advertised that we were starting a group for carers, patients and bereaved people. The first evening, one lady stood up and said 'well, if there's nothing else that I've learned tonight, when I go home and tuck my husband in bed, I shan't be doing it alone, all of you will be doing that as well – and that gives me a lot of support'. It is small things like that that actually help them.

We started it with two therapists and the first day, two people arrived. Six years on, we've got five therapists, we do it twice a month and, on average, sixty to seventy people come. They can meet people experiencing the same type of things as themselves. We don't turn anybody away.

Counsellor 2

There are also many specific therapies available both for people coming in for the day and for those staying in the hospice:

They come in and talk to one of the nurses about their medication, how they feel, have their blood pressure taken and then we have about five or six kinds of massage – reflexology, Reiki, chiropody, head-massage and all that. They just put their names down and they get seen to.

Volunteer 1

If people have got really bad anxiety, I might do a relaxation session. I use all different techniques. It could be progressive relaxation where they lie comfortably and you play soft music and you get them to tense up their toes and relax, and then move up through the whole body. Or other relaxation where it's more imagery, so imagine walking down a beach and hearing the waves and the wind and the birds. I don't do it that often, but I enjoy it.

Occupational therapist

The word 'therapy' is a Greek word, meaning 'to be with'. Often, it's being with someone that is very important. Within the therapy session, there is very rarely much talking going on. What happens, certainly with the day care patients, is that once they're in the therapy room, they can switch off, they start to relax and unwind. The shoulder or whatever it is you're working on may have been the catalyst at one point, but very often, it's the knowledge that that's their space.

I practise adapted massage, reflexology, Reiki and spiritual healing. The treatments are adapted to the individual. Not all therapists would agree with me, but here, the treatment is a form of comforting, it's giving somebody choice, it's touch that isn't task orientated – it's about people feeling good about themselves.

Complementary therapist

Or counselling:

Counselling is all about being with that person and try to get an understanding of their frame of reference. Obviously, with terminally ill people, you are not making it better, you are making it calm and pain free – but emotionally, you can't always fix the mind. Nurses tend to want patients to have all the conflicts in their life resolved. But we have limited time, because either people are in here for a week's respite or symptom control or they are terminally ill and are only here a short while. So you have to judge what you can get done in that time without unravelling someone's whole past – you haven't got time to get that tidy.

Counsellor 1

Hospice compared to hospital care

Hospices are seen to be very different than hospitals. Different people notice different aspects:

They're a lot more relaxed about the washing here. In the NHS, there is a whole thing of everyone has to be washed and the bed has to be made – that goes back to when matrons were around. Here, it's a lot about what the patient wants to do. If one of our patients said that they'd prefer to have a bath later, fine, I'm here all day, I can give him a Jacuzzi later, not a problem. They really love the Jacuzzi. There's a chair they sit on and we can hoist them down and then push the button and away you go.

Senior staff nurse 4

Patients are basically trapped – once you are diagnosed, you get caught up in the health service and all your choices are taken away. You get told 'you need chemotherapy, radiotherapy, drugs'. And for food, in hospital it is 'here is the soup – take it or leave it'. But I go in and say 'here are your choices for what to eat today', they can pick something. It may seem a small option, but to the patient, it is a big option, as they have grabbed a bit of control.

You think this could be this person's last meal – you want it to be nice, you don't want it to be just run of the mill. When you are doing a hundred meals, by the time you serve the hundredth one, it's not going to be as fresh, as it has cooked slightly longer. But here, everything is direct from the kitchen to the patients – it is as good as you have created it. I think that makes a difference.

Chef

I've had experience of hospital lately, because my mother-in-law was a patient. I've watched how nurses work – and I do feel that we are more attentive to people. We listen more, we're listening to the unsaid things. My mother-in-law complained that there wasn't staff around. We're here for people – that's the main difference. Even when we're busy, it's a small environment and patients see it as that. If they want to ask you something, they know where to find you.

Senior staff nurse 2

People who are dying can be angry – angry with the medical profession for not diagnosing quickly enough, angry with other members of the family who haven't got involved in their care. But after working in the NHS where people were really quick to complain, I found it doesn't happen here. It is a completely different ethos. That was one of the first things I noticed – nobody was thundering about saying 'I know my patient's rights – I want this, I want that'. Here nobody asks for anything. Everybody says this is nothing like a hospital and then ask 'why can't everywhere be like this?' We have only a small number of patients and it is just pure care. And we are the same team more or less every day.

Counsellor 1

There is particular concern about the way people die in hospital:

In the hospital, people who were terminally ill died on an open ward. They had no privacy and it affected other patients on the ward. If you've got a lot of family crying around a bed, you don't need to be Einstein to realise that this person is dying. If the chap in the next bed is ready for discharge and you've got all these people very sad and crying, it's a bit like 'well, don't laugh, because my father's dying' – it's not an ideal place.

Nurse 2

A few people have experience of working in a hospital:

I spent ten years in the NHS. You tried to do your best, but that was very much a struggled best in that there were so many shortages in resources. You often finished a shift being quite upset and frustrated that you couldn't do more. Coming here, although we are very busy at the moment, we are able to give more time to the patients and to the relatives.

Senior staff nurse 4

I got quite disillusioned working in the NHS. I did a couple of nights on a geriatric ward and this lady came in very late. She was a lovely lady, she had her hair done, her nails were painted, makeup on. She took a lot of a care in herself, so I asked if she normally liked to wash before getting into bed and she said 'oh yes, please!' I got her a bowl and I was told off for it – 'we don't do that'. I was then told something like 'don't give her a bowl to wash herself – they'll all want one'. I think they got so stuck in their routine, they didn't allow themselves to be flexible.

Senior staff nurse 1

And, on occasion, this disillusionment could have large consequences:

I was in charge of the ward and we'd had a gentleman die and his wife was beside the bed – they'd been married 64 years. I didn't rush him off the ward. I got called to the Director of Nursing and was told off, 'do you not know it is the middle of winter and there is a bed crisis?' I was supposed to get another patient in that bed as soon as possible. I just said to him 'well, do you not know that you've just lost a nurse?' This poor woman, how could you shoo her away from someone who she's spent her whole adult life with? I was not prepared to do it, so I had to give my notice there and then.

Sister

What is special about a hospice

The sense that hospices feel special underlies many of the things people say about working in them. Nurses and other staff take enormous pride in their hospice:

There's something wonderful about a hospice. It's part of the caring. Everybody says the same. It's a happy atmosphere, because the nurses are cheerful and they feel appreciated – good work does engender a good spirit. Like people who go out to these places in Africa – when they're interviewed, they're always terribly positive.

Chaplain 1

You need professionalism for what you're dealing with here. The suddenness of death. Someone might come in here in an ambulance at 9.00 in the morning and be dead by 12.00 – you just need that professionalism to help you cope with it. They've absolutely mastered it here, it's all done calmly and smoothly.

Healthcare assistant 2

In my generation, people looked after each other, particularly working-class people. They use a highly-overused word, 'community'. But community pre-war meant your grandmother living round the corner and your sister and her husband and eight kids living up the road, everybody pulled together. This is really what happens here – everybody pulls together. If somebody doesn't feel well, one of the other patients will go and have a chat with them, put their arm round them and just have a talk. The care and attention that one gets is wonderful. If I were sick, I would think there was no greater place in the world that you can go to than here.

Volunteer 1

There is an effort to make a hospice not seem like an institution. This can be seen in the degree of flexibility:

Pets are allowed in. It's really nice. Obviously, patients are going to miss their pets, they're going to worry about them. Different people worry about different things. You've got to find out what's bothering them, prioritise what they want and what they need and then go from there.

Senior staff nurse 1

Sometimes, you may actually give somebody a wash at seven in the evening, because if you go to them in the morning and they are feeling really poorly and they say they don't feel like it now, that's fine. It is not a hospital. The way we work is that they tell us what they need.

Healthcare assistant 1

We have a patient at the moment who's been very angry, but today he's coming out of it, because we are giving him time, sitting with him, talking to him. He thought he was in a prisoner of war camp. He kept saying that he's seen the line and he can't cross it – the line is the skirting board, and he feels that he can't cross that. I've taken him for a walk, 'come on, we'll cross the line together, because there is no line, you're just imagining it' and just helping him talk, show that we listen. He's a bundle of joy today and it's lovely to see him.

Healthcare assistant 2

It can also be seen in the particular thoughtfulness of staff:

Patients want a place that is as much like home as possible, but where they get medical care. So work clothes, like a white coat, would make it a bit formal. We wear ordinary clothes – we don't wear white coats. The nurses wear a uniform, but it's not something that would intimidate patients or make them feel it's a hospital. It's not too starchy.

Doctor 2

We have discovered that a big plate of food freaks patients and puts them off food altogether. We have bought side plates, to deceive the eye. For soup bowls, we use the little bowls that you get rice in, in a Chinese restaurant – there might only be about three tablespoons of soup in it, but because they finish it, the patient goes 'God, I didn't think I would eat all that!' It is just an optical illusion.

They might have one thin slice of roast beef and a very small Yorkshire pudding, one Brussels sprout and two pieces of fresh carrot for colour and maybe one boiled or roast potato. And then we serve a dessert. So they are actually getting a meal, but it's like a little kid's meal – but to them, it looks like they have eaten a whole Sunday roast dinner. And they finish it, because it is not that much – they can always ask for more if they want to. We have worked out, through talking to them every day, that that's what they're happy with.

Chef

Volunteers take menu orders for patients – everything is ordered individually. They also keep the place looking decent, fill the flower vases up, chat to people and serve lunch. In the afternoon, they offer tea and maybe do extra things for people. What the volunteers offer is a kind of rota of normal people coming in and out, who aren't your distressed family, who aren't nurses or doctors. It's tremendously important to people. They comment all the time on how nice it is to see volunteers.

Volunteer coordinator

Attention is given to the whole person:

It's being able to practise medicine in a holistic way, where you do look at physical symptoms, but also the social, spiritual, psychological care of the patient. A surgeon just wants to go there, cut it off – and that's it. But someone's got to be there when the patient comes round – look at the pain, how are they feeling, how are they going to cope at home? That's what palliative care's about, not just the problem there, but other things relating to it. You have time to care for the patient as a person, not as a case – it's more humane, it's more down-to-earth.

Doctor 2

I don't know whether what we do prolongs life, but I think we make for a better quality of life. Every day, you see a patient who is eating and think 'you have got a bit of colour, you are more lucid, you are sitting up, you are doing normal-ish things'. I tell patients 'just think of yourself as a car – if you don't put petrol in that car, it won't run. If you don't put some sort of food in there, you will sleep – your family will be sitting here and you will miss a lot of time when you could be talking to them'. Then they will agree to try some breakfast. And because they eat, whether it is physical or psychological, they do have a sort of 'up' day. It is partly about how it is perceived. You can see the family are worried sick about the person who is dying, but when they see them eating, they think 'oh, she is eating!' The patient then sees the relief in their family's face. So they feed off each other. That's what I am trying to achieve – just bringing that little level of quality of life back.

Chef

The needs of families are taken into account:

This is the place where families matter, where spiritual aspects – not just religious beliefs, but lifting one's spirits and emotions – matter, where the whole package is looked at. It's a truly holistic approach. You could say it's at the cutting edge, because this is the place where a lot of things are learned, so in that sense it's a vanguard of where healthcare is going.

Volunteer 2

Most people want to die in their own home. But because it puts pressure on the family, it gets complicated. You see husbands and wives and they are not husband and wife – they are patient and carer. By coming in here, they can let us be the carers and regain that relationship of husband and wife. People sometimes say 'I didn't want to come here, but actually I feel safe now that I am here'. I can't say that everyone is 100% happy, but most of them are. When we see families the day after the death, they say 'this place is amazing, you have been so helpful' – we rarely hear anything else.

Counsellor 1

And everything is very much led by what patients want:

My aim is to give people peace at the end of their life. If patients want to open up and discuss things or even have a cry, whatever they want to do is fine by me. If they want to give me a cuddle, I will cuddle them. I am quite tactile and there is a warmth about the place, which people always comment on. There are no boundaries as far as I am concerned. So if at the end of someone's life, I can give them peace and comfort and help the families to make their passing easier, even if it is a tiny way, then I feel that I have done a good job. And when I leave here of a night-time, I need to know that I have given 110%.

Healthcare assistant 1

I see myself as helping people to live until they die. You try and improve their quality of life as much as you can until they die. It's very client centred – you're really led by what the patient is needing at that moment in time.

I might go in to someone's home with an idea of assessing if they can get out of bed onto a chair or get on and off the toilet. A lot of patients do find it quite difficult, so it's just looking at different devices to make it easier for them to do things on their own. Maybe a raised toilet seat might mean that they can go to the toilet independently. But maybe the patient had a really awful night, they might value it more if you just chatted to them for fifteen minutes.

Occupational therapist

Everything that happens in the day centre is led by the needs and wishes of the clients. And that creates a very different relationship with the service because it's not being imposed on them. We have quarterly 'business meetings' looking at the business of providing the service, where I sit down with people who come to the centre and talk about what's going well, what's not going well, what they want next, what they want to be developed further. When we first held meetings, the two things that people came up with was that they'd like more complementary therapies and complained about the food. So that told me people didn't feel nurtured. I recruited additional complementary therapists. I also asked what the clients didn't like about the food and when they saw that there were changes based on what they had asked for I think it gave them a sense of being heard and supported.

Day centre manager

Staff often take on whatever role is needed:

I'm not as hands-on clinically any more, but I've not lost my skills and I'm keen not to lose them. Today, patient dependency is quite high and there's a lot going on, so I just had to help out. We're a team and no one is more important than the other, so we all help each other. I helped with doling out the meals because that was something that needed to be done. It's doing whatever lightens the load of the team and helps the patients.

Head nurse

Patients can be so surprised when a sister dishes up their meal. They look at your badge and say 'a sister's just served me!' And they actually feel quite privileged. A sister giving them a wash, they think they're special. New staff as well – they get very shocked that the sister is there putting on a pair of gloves.

Sister

The importance of this time in a person's life is compared to birth:

The way I look at it, you get one shot at this. It's the same as midwifery – it's not like you can go back and do it again. They die once and you have to get it right. You can't sit there and say 'I'm sorry, I got that a bit wrong, can we do that again?' What you do, these relatives will remember for the rest of their lives. If you cock up or if you come across wrong at all, that is what they're going to carry with them. It can be a heavy responsibility.

Sister

A good death is very important. Coming into this world and leaving this world are momentous occasions – I've been privileged to see both ends of the spectrum. People fear death so much in this society that whatever we can do to make that less fearful for patients and their relatives and friends is really important.

Senior staff nurse 2

PART I

THE WORK UNDERTAKEN

CHAPTER 2

The nature of the work

Hospices are busy organisations with many different types of activities going on. There is, of course, a lot of work with patients and relatives, but also all sorts of 'back-room' activities, such as administrative tasks and staff management. This chapter explores the day-to-day work of a hospice, including the provision of day care and working with patients at home.

The rhythm of a day

The best way of capturing a snapshot of life in a hospice is to listen to people describing their day. Most nurses say that they begin with a handover and then set about working with patients:

> We have a handover for all patients in the hospice which we all sit in on – that usually lasts about half an hour. We then come up and allocate the patients to the staff for the washes, so that we know who's going to wash whom. Then I would give out the medications. While I'm doing that, I'm also assessing patients. Maybe I've never met them before, maybe I left at 10.00 pm last night and I'll see a deterioration. If it's someone who's dying, the relatives will be there and I'll talk to them about how they felt the patient was in the night. If there's things that need organising, we talk to the doctors, noting which patients have deteriorated or what might need to be changed.
>
> The patients who are dying have a 'sub-cut driver', a 24-hour pump, which might have a sedative or other drugs to dry up excess secretions. We check those at every drug round, to ensure that the pumps are running properly. If we feel a patient has particular pain or they're more agitated than they should be, we change the syringe and increase the drug. Some have other medications, such as relaxants or anti-retrovirals for the HIV patients. Elderly people may have heart or other conditions, so they'll have all the medications they take anyway, as well as for the disease they're in here with.
>
> Once medication is done and everyone's been washed, it's lunchtime and then the afternoon is just spent with us generally making sure everyone's happy, relatives are all up to date and happy here. Everyone's pain free, everyone is as comfortable as we can possibly get them, until the night staff come on.
>
> *Senior staff nurse 4*

Starting out, patients are fed – either helped to be fed or they are set up to feed themselves. They are then allocated to nurses and healthcare assistants for the day. The things we need to do would be administering medication and providing personal hygiene – washing and shaving, that kind of stuff. Patients are not able to do it so effectively when they are dying, so they need help. Coordinating everything, such as physiotherapists, if needed. Then perhaps dealing with undertakers, the paperwork around death. A lot of it is assessing what the patient needs and what the families need in terms of bereavement – whether they will need counselling or not. If so, we refer them to our social workers.

Staff nurse

We start work at 7.30. When we come in, we have the handover. The night staff hand over the shift from the previous night. Each patient has a folder and the doctor's notes, so we go through those folders and we see what their needs are. Maybe somebody is unable to stand, so before we go in to them, we would have to know that they need a hoist, so that you don't say 'come on, Mrs. Jones, up you get' and she lands on the floor! We have our allocated patients. We could have nine or ten, or we could have six who are very heavily dependent. We are hands-on with the patients. In a way, we are the ears and eyes of the place, because if we come in and see a big change from the previous day, it is for us to say that to a trained nurse, so that they realise and a doctor can be alerted.

Then we go and greet all the patients. We sit them up, we get them comfortable and if they need their dentures put in, if they need to use the toilet, if some are too unwell then we let them sleep. The food comes down from the kitchen area. Some patients may need feeding and maybe somebody can't even hold their own glass, so we would spend time with them. Once breakfast is over, we have a break where we go and have a coffee and something to eat.

And then what I call the 'real care' starts. One of my patients might be terminally ill and they would need their position changed more than somebody who's independent or needs minimal assistance. So we have to assess which patients are priority. And we go and give our care. We are not timed on how long we spend with a patient. If we need to spend an hour and a half with somebody, either because of the hands-on situation or because they are in a dreadful state emotionally, we can do that. We know that we don't have to walk away from somebody.

The afternoon is generally quieter. Quite often after lunch, they have a rest. But because the bulk of the hands-on care is done in the morning, the afternoon can be many things. We have admissions, we have people going home – and also a big part of the job is the families.

Healthcare assistant 1

When I come in first thing in the morning – I'm renowned for this – they say I've 'got a face on'. What it is, I'm planning my day. I am a bit of a control freak – once I know what's happening and who's going to be doing what, I'm happy. I chill out, I laugh and joke, but for that first half an hour or so, I'm very tunnelled into getting my priorities set. You never know what to expect. Anything can change even between 7.30 and 10.00 in the morning, I might have to totally change the priorities I'd set. So it's constantly being able to look at the wider picture. As sisters, we do exactly the same as staff nurses do. Today, I've done two bed baths. I've never been able to do that anywhere else.

Sister

Particular roles

But nurses and nursing staff are not the only ones who work with patients. Others have more particular roles, keeping the hospice going and attending to the needs of patients:

We start at 7.30 in the morning and straight away it is go and collect the old water jugs from the previous evening. We get them washed and supply fresh glasses with iced water. We then go back to the kitchen, look at what the patients have requested for that day and start preparing. For breakfast, they have a choice of porridge or cereals and they can also have a cooked breakfast – bacon, mushrooms, tomatoes, sausages, fried bread, and poached, scrambled, or fried eggs, all those common breakfast things, grapefruit segments and prunes.

We serve the patients and then we come back to the kitchen for staff breakfasts and then we start cooking lunch. About 10.00, we start getting all our ingredients ready. We supply two choices, but we also have a vegetarian choice and we also do things like rolls with fillings, prawn cocktails, salads and baked potatoes. We serve lunch at 1.00 and that can last till about 2.00 and we then go back to the kitchen, the girls wash up all the trolley stuff and I go with my menu and ask what they would like for the next day.

For supper, we make something light, like maybe an omelette, grilled fish, sandwiches. That goes round at 5.30 or so. Then during the evening, the nurses and the carers have got access to the catering department, so if somebody says they would like some toast and marmalade, they can just go in the kitchen, make the toast and take it to the patient. Even though the kitchen officially closes at 7.00, it is never really closed – there is always something, whether it is a sandwich or some cornflakes.

Chef

My work is very much practicalities. The first thing I do every morning is check my diary. I came in Monday morning and three people had died over the weekend, so then there was a note what time their next of kin are coming in to see me to collect the death certificate. We stagger the times that the families come in, because if you have three families turning up at the same time, they can get upset at some point and that all takes time. You need to be very methodical. They've got an appointment with me. I make sure that I have got the death certificate completed, I check valuables to see if they've got anything in the safe, I would have any property ready, so by the time the next of kin arrives it's all set up. I simply bring them in here with the certificate and all the patient's worldly goods and then I start to explain what the family have to do now, which is mainly to register the death.

Nothing can really happen until the death has been registered. So you've got to make sure that everything's done quickly and efficiently. In general, it's about four or five days. Anyone who dies here has to register with the local council here. That's often shocked people, because they think that they will register where they lived. The registry office has an emergency number should they be required at the weekend.

Patient affairs officer

And others will be focused on administrative issues, such as admissions and discharges:

My job is looking at the criteria for coming into the hospice, whether it's an appropriate admission both medically and financially. We have contracts with health authorities and we need to check that they're in the right health authority and yes, they might have cancer but what are they actually coming in here for? I have to have a referral form from someone, like a consultant, district nurse or social worker – a relative cannot refer you here. Once I get that referral, I'll be in contact with someone, such as hospital staff if they're in hospital, to have an update on their medical condition. I'm responsible for making sure that it's an appropriate place for a patient who's coming in.

Discharge nurse 2

I establish rapport with patients by introducing myself early on. I explain that I am the discharge coordinator, but that doesn't mean they are going home. I then say that I will be in touch with them in a couple of days to see what I can do to help. I try to make it clear that I am on their side, because if you are sick and you have been having problems at home and somebody starts talking about your going home, it can be frightening.

I need to be sensitive to what each person wants. Some are keen to go home. I then need to tell the district nurse that they want their independence, but to please keep a check on them. I will never say to somebody that they are not fit enough to go home. The hardest ones are those where, because of their disease, their understanding is impaired, such as patients with brain tumours. There was a patient recently who was determined that she would go home and would cope, but we were worried about her safety in case of a fall. I would never force somebody, because that isn't my decision. Luckily, a relative stepped forward and said they would take on the care – we will lay on extra back-up care as much as possible.

Discharge nurse 1

Day patients

In another part of the hospice, there will be people working with patients who come in for day care of one kind or another:

> We have separate programmes for cancer patients and HIV patients, but we've always encouraged people to use the service in the way that they want. Some of our HIV clients have an immense difficulty with other people knowing their status, so they can come to our cancer care days. The two groups share a lot of the same problems, symptoms and issues. They are an incredibly supportive community, in terms of helping each other with difficult life situations, yet coming from very different communities, age groups and ethnic backgrounds. People feel welcomed here. Some people in the cancer care programme are in recovery and can become inspirational to others. They can also become advocates for others, who may have lost a sense of themselves because they are so consumed by their diagnosis or treatment that they lose hope.

Day centre manager

> I work in the day centre. I come in usually just after 9.00 in the mornings and leave about 2.00, unless there's a concert on and then I stay a bit longer, because it's quite good fun. Another volunteer is usually here already and we start laying the tables. There's always flowers on the table, placemats, serviettes, wine glasses and ordinary drinking glasses. Gradually, the patients start coming in – some of them haven't spoken with anyone apart from the Macmillan nurse, for quite a few days. A lot of these people are on their own – we give them a cup of tea and a biscuit and chat. We talk about what's been on the television, what's been in the newspapers, just to make them feel at home and gradually the place fills up, because we have volunteer drivers who bring people in, apart from the ambulances which go round to pick them up. We average about 26 people. And we make everybody welcome, have a laugh, I warn them that unless they enjoy themselves, they're going to get hit.
>
> In the late morning, a physiotherapist comes in and most people take part in the exercises. She starts off with deep breathing and then chair exercises, just to make you more mobile, make you breathe better, how to relax your eyes and generally to make you feel good. Afterwards, we bring out balloons and put some old-fashioned music on and they punch balloons up and down and have a fabulous time. We have an excellent lunch,

soup or melon, main course and delightful desserts – they sit down and the volunteers serve them their lunch. Wine and all kinds of drinks.

Volunteer 1

Some help with spiritual or practical needs:

I come in once a week to the day centre and I have a little communion service for the Catholic patients. I chat with them and then I will go round to see if there are any others. I don't have contact with patients of other denominations.

Chaplain 1

One week I focus on day care patients and the following week I focus on in-patients. Day care patients arrive at 10.00 am. It's their day out – they may have made a lot of effort to get dressed up and come out. You look round the room and everybody looks 'normal', completely fit and well. They arrive, have a cup of tea, chat and then usually I do about three treatments in the morning and the same in the afternoon. They are just short treatments – maybe a gentle foot or shoulder massage. Some people have a short treatment, their lunch, then maybe something else, such as a manicure.

You have to be very aware of knowing when you need to pass information on to someone. If somebody is not breathing so well, you might ask if they have mentioned it to a nurse or the doctor or if they would mind if you mentioned it to someone, 'I'll just have a little word with the nurse for you about it, it will put my mind at rest'. You have to be very professional, because sometimes people want to mask things and pretend that they're fine.

Complementary therapist

On an ordinary day, I might go up to the day centre and help somebody apply for benefits. We do a huge amount of work around welfare rights, because we have a lot of patients with a very low income – or, if they're asylum seekers, no income. We also do a lot of work helping people to access housing and other services. So there can be a huge emphasis on practical work. This morning, I was on the phone to somebody who I'm helping get money for a washing machine. He has HIV and gets a lot of night sweats, he really needs a washer-drier, but he's long term unemployed, so I've been writing to different charities to try and get him one.

Social worker

The hospice at night

Hospices seem to feel very different at night, generally more peaceful:

At night, the hospice is generally quieter, because our main concern is trying to get everyone relaxed so they have a peaceful sleep. When they wake up in the morning, they need to be having as good a day as possible, because they need to have quality time with their families and friends. So it's really important that they have a good night's sleep.

Senior staff nurse 4

It's different here at night. Very quiet most of the time, very peaceful. The staff have more time to talk with patients. A lot of patients will be asleep and there will be the odd one who can't sleep and you go and sit and chat to them or make them a drink. So it's different. It's not got the buzz and the business – and that's when people start to think and when they're more frightened. So you'll find lights being switched on and cups of tea being made and you try to put their worries to bed.

Head of hospice 1

Indeed, some find it a bit too peaceful:

I prefer days. You haven't got to keep quiet so much. You can have a laugh, because everybody's awake and you can sit out in the sunshine with them. You're more involved, because they're more awake. Whereas night-time, some of them just go to sleep and they're out for the count all night.

Healthcare assistant 2

It is also a time when some deep discussions can go on:

One of the nice things about night duty is that you have time to listen to people talk. You don't have the telephones, you don't have people coming and going, you don't have quite so much administrative activity. You will have more time for people – listening time or just being there time.

Relatives can stay if they want. They will tend to stay if the patient has asked them to. They will also stay if they anticipate things are not going to be good or because they know time is limited and they won't have many more nights to be with that person. For whatever reason, we will encourage them to stay if they want to. You hear about what they are facing and you try to help prepare them. Quite often, they just want to talk.

Senior staff nurse 2

At night, there is less rush to do things. The night nurses have their break time when they can rest, but they check on patients regularly. And some-times the patients, when they're lonely and scared, will open up and they tell the night staff things. That's when we get an insight into their psycho-logical problems, their social or spiritual problems – it helps in the holistic management of the patient.

Doctor 2

But patients can also have greater needs at night:

> Patients over the years have said the nights are the worst time, because if they can't sleep, they feel like they are the only person who is awake and they are lying there with this illness and the fear and not knowing what's going to happen. So the nights can be particularly stressful.
>
> *Healthcare assistant 1*

> There was a young man who was in the Falkland's War and he developed problems with flashbacks. He would see snipers in his room at night – he would wake up sweating, shouting out and, of course, he'd been dreaming. The nurses tried to spend time with him, not making the room dark and then discussing with the doctors what type of medication could perhaps help him.
>
> *Nurse 2*

> A few patients find it difficult to sleep, they get scared to get into bed in case they pass away and will sit or sleep in a chair. They will look at the bed and go 'I am not getting in there' – they will only get in there if they are really, really ill. But if they are just sitting in a chair, their bottom is going to get very sore, so you try and coax them in, 'if we get you into bed, you will be able to stretch out and turn onto your side, it will be a lot better' and then you get them in and they go 'God, I should have done this ages ago'.
>
> *Nurse 1*

Patients at home

Looking after patients at home brings its own set of issues. There is less control over the home environment and less certainty that someone will always be there to help:

> It was very scary at first. About three months after I started, I set up a syringe driver for a patient who was dying at home. In hospital, you can always go back and check it and adjust it, so for me to leave it was quite distressing. I was worried about what would happen – one of my colleagues said she had the same reaction. The next day I phoned the wife, just to see how the night went and she said he was all right. That was reassuring. I had been worried that he'd died and it would be my fault, even though I knew that's not the case. If someone is going to die, they're going to die – my interventions won't matter. That was hard.
>
> You learn to pre-empt things, to have things ready or in the home – medications, extra care from the district nurses, the GPs. You're getting everybody on board. I can see signs of deteriorating health very much easier now. I like to be able to prepare as much as I can.
>
> *Community nurse*

You never really know what to expect when you go into a patient's home. Sometimes you will speak to someone and you think it's going to be a bit unclean and you get there and it's really lovely and clean. Once, I went into someone's home and it was very cluttered and dirty – there were newspapers from the 1960s piled up on the staircase, which was dangerous in itself, and plastic bags and bags of clothes. I was quite distressed that she'd been living there all those years. But she didn't think there was anything wrong with it. I went into the kitchen – there was a big bucket of live meal worms in it – when I asked why, she said she used to have a bird and these were for it. You'd like to go home and shower, but I've got to go back to work – there's a report to do and you need to make sure the patient has settled back in.

Occupational therapist

Patients have strong views about what they want in the home and how they want to be:

I see a lot of people at home in their own environment. There are many different jobs in the home – for instance, assessing people for a wheelchair and then showing them how to go up and down the street or on and off the kerb. Or seeing if they can independently make a cup of tea. Things that we take for granted are sometimes quite important.

I try to set people up to be as comfortable as possible and as independent as they can be. No one likes for their independence to be taken away. You've got to be very careful to observe the atmosphere, because some people will feel quite hostile about having equipment in their home. A commode next to the bed could be awful. It's quite tricky, because you might think this person really needs to have a particular bit of equipment, but they don't want it. I've learned to say, 'often, people find that this is quite useful' or I take a catalogue with pictures. I also say this is something they could try for a week or so, they don't have to keep it forever. If they don't want it, it can be taken away. But then, you get patients who say 'can I have a wheelchair?' 'Can I have a cushion?' Some people want a lot and others don't want anything – it's usually the ones who really need the things that try not to have them and the ones that don't really need the things are always eager to.

Occupational therapist

It takes skill to be sensitive to a variety of needs:

I've had situations where people don't want me in, because they feel they're not dying. They'll ask why I am there, 'well I'm here to advise you on your symptoms – your pain control and your nausea. I'm not here because you're dying.' People sometimes ask whether they should have treatment. I'd be honest with them and explain what would happen if they have it or not, but that I don't know how long they have. And then I would

ask how they want their life to be. It's giving them the options and allowing them to say they don't want to be in and out of hospitals with
infections, but would rather have their last few months being well. It's
giving them the opportunity to talk about it. I'm someone who's removed
from their family, so they can be honest about how they feel.

Community nurse

You become more sensitive to different cultures and adjust to it. Muslims
don't always like to have carers coming in – they prefer their family to be
doing personal care and the domestic things. If you don't know, you just
ask them, 'is it appropriate for me to do this?' and they will tell you. For
example, if I wanted to check the range of movement on a Muslim gentleman's knee, I would first ask 'may I touch your leg?' And sometimes
Jewish men don't like shaking your hand. I used to introduce myself and
stick my hand out, but once, the person just nodded and I thought OK.
You learn from that and change what you do.

Occupational therapist

There can also be circumstances where it is very difficult for people to manage at
home:

I had to see someone who was living on a boat. It was a big learning curve
but also very frustrating, because he was deteriorating quite rapidly and it
was difficult to get up on to the boat. I couldn't put any steps there, I
couldn't put a rail up. Inside, the boat was very narrow. There just wasn't
the space for things to lift the mattress up and down on the bed. I was
problem solving and asking for advice from other occupational therapists
– all the things we came up with just weren't suitable.

We try and accommodate the patient's wishes. The patient was admitted to hospital and got an infection and then he came to the hospice – the
idea was that maybe he would go back to the boat. Both he and his wife
were kind of in denial as well, so that made it quite difficult, 'maybe in a
week's time, I'll be able to walk and I'll be able to go up the steps' – and
he wasn't even on his feet. There was a lot of work for all of us involved,
just trying to make them realise that he might not be able to walk and
giving them alternatives. If he really wanted to go, I would have tried to
adapt the boat, even if it was just for one night.

Occupational therapist

Sometimes, a person returning home can fall apart – people go home and
after a couple of days, reality kicks in and they are not coping. They then
need someone in to help them. I have had only two gentlemen come back.
One had a stroke and had come in for respite, but when he went home he
became suddenly much less well, so we brought him back within 24 hours.
The other wasn't really fit for discharge, but insisted that he wanted to go

home – that fell apart within a day and we got him back in Normally, we can pinpoint those and will deliberately hold the bed or three days – we will tell the family that we know that he might have problems and to feel free to bring them back.

Discharge nurse 1

Managing the hospice

Finally, there are managerial responsibilities for staff. As in many organisations, this means ensuring that everything is ticking over as it should and everyone feels supported:

I have one-to-one meetings with the people I directly manage as well as with our consultant. I like to be kept abreast of what's happening. I like to support the staff and I don't particularly like a problem to happen, if it could have been averted. I don't want to know all the ins and outs of everything – I just want to know if there's a potential problem, so we can work with each other to try and either minimise it or be prepared for it.

Head of hospice 2

I'm sort of middle management, so my role is to coordinate the health care assistants and the other staff nurses on the wards. On some occasions, I would be the nurse in charge, responsible for all the patients and the visitors who are in the hospice at the time – and responsible for their care and administration of medication. We try as much as we can to do hands-on nursing, but often I'm in the treatment room dispensing medication.

Senior staff nurse 1

In addition to supporting the patients, I support the more junior members of staff. I'm the coordinator of the shift for the day, 7.30 till 9.00, ensuring that it runs as smoothly as possible, everyone's supported as much as possible and that all the patients are receiving the appropriate care.

Senior staff nurse 4

I see as many of the volunteers as I can every week, because I think one of the main parts of my job is for them to have somebody they can come to if there's a problem. Volunteers need support and recognition for what they're doing. The nursing staff and doctors may be too busy to say thank you. So that's an important part of my job, supporting them and organising their rotas.

Volunteer coordinator

Those who manage staff often learn how to do so with sensitivity:

I will play to people's needs. With one person, I can be very straightforward and pull them up on something, but with another that might start a full-scale hysteria attack, so I would dumb down and say 'I don't know if it was me, but do you think this is right?' I learned a lot of from watching the first ward manager that I worked for here – she sussed out very quickly people's strengths and weaknesses and what approach was going to work.

Sister

Such work can also mean ensuring that standards are maintained:

When I come on duty, the first thing I do – I do it surreptitiously, but they all know I do it – is to check everybody. I check that they're wearing the right uniform and that they're as professional as they should be. Because if I don't pick it up, somebody else will.

Head nurse

And there are plenty of meetings of one kind or another:

There are several meetings in the hospice. We have a head of department meeting and that's partly peer supervision, where we talk about particular problems, or it's making some decisions. There's a management team, which are the managers of each department. If there are any particular issues, such as ensuring that doors are locked when staff leave, we take it there and they disseminate it to their various departments. We have a meeting every morning, where we'll discuss any changes overnight in each patient's condition. And once a week, we have a discharge meeting where we will discuss potential discharges. There's ad hoc meetings between nurses and doctors as well.

Head nurse

Multi-disciplinary team meetings are important in palliative care, where every member of the team gets together and has a say. It is very much a holistic approach, where you have the physiotherapist, social worker, dietician, volunteer coordinator and everyone has a chance to speak if they feel the need. I think everyone listens and values other people's input.

Doctor 1

CHAPTER 3

Responding to patients and relatives

The broad day-to-day work of a hospice has now been described. In this chapter, the more detailed aspects of working with patients and relatives are explored.

Welcoming and reassuring

Clearly, a lot of the day-to-day work revolves around patients in one way or another. Part of this is just providing them with some company and a sense of reassurance:

> Lots of patients and families are really frightened of coming here. Part of our job is to greet them at the door – and you can see the absolute terror on their face. So we will hold their hands, give human contact and just be compassionate. They just want you to treat them normally, give them some normality back. They don't want to keep talking about cancer and dying. They may have been ill for some time and they often say 'it is so nice to have a laugh' – because everybody who comes to visit them asks 'how are you?' 'Have you got pain?' They forget that they want to talk about the normal things 'what's Tony Blair up to this week?'
>
> *Healthcare assistant 1*

> We sit and talk with patients. That's a big part of the day. I think it's essential, especially when the patient is very depressed. We get them to come out of that grey area and try to make them laugh or talk about the old days. I talk about everything, and it helps them a great deal.
>
> *Healthcare assistant 2*

> A little rule that I've made for myself is I will not finish an encounter with someone unless I can walk away feeling I've left them feeling better in some way or other. I'm sure there are times you don't, but I'll stick it out and use humour when all else fails. People are all human and you can always find a soft part in somebody. If you can't make people feel that they've gained something or they're happier, then you haven't achieved anything. Even if it's breaking the worst news ever, you've got to find a twist and finish on an up beat. You leave some element of hope.
>
> *Consultant*

Occasionally, new staff can do the wrong thing:

> One day, when I hadn't been here long, the undertakers came to the door, and they'd brought some flowers. You could tell they were flowers from a funeral. I went around to the back door and the guy was really sweet and said 'there's an awful lot, love, let me help you, I'll take them through'. I thought he was helping me. But he had a big tall hat on, with the black velvet ribbons at the back, and he's traipsing through the hospice with his flowers – I didn't think! One of the nurses explained that people from the cemeteries were not allowed to come through the hospice, because it could upset the patients. I said 'I'm ever so sorry, he just followed me'. I had put my foot in it!
>
> *Senior staff nurse 1*

Physical and practical needs

But part of this involvement is trying to gauge patients' needs. This may be for particular physical problems:

> Sometimes, I'll say to the consultants, 'I don't know what's wrong, but there's something today, he's not right' and they will keep an eye out. A lot of the nurses here nurse with their instincts. You just know that there's something not right, but you don't know what, so you just have to wait until something comes out.
>
> *Sister*

> A big bugbear for me is mouth care – sometimes it can get forgotten. You will go into a patient and they will look lovely, they will have had their hair washed, they will have had a bath and they go to speak and you say 'put your tongue out' and they have got little sores and nobody has actually thought to do that. I find it a bit frustrating that other people aren't as up on that as I would like them to be. But on the whole it is excellent, people will brush their teeth and all the rest of it.
>
> *Healthcare assistant 1*

> Patients can be very demanding sometimes, but I try and find out why. I ask what's wrong, starting at the head and working down to the foot. You can usually get something out of them and say, 'A-ha! I'll get you something for it'. I find it upsetting when patients come in from hospital in a terrible state. We had a guy in the other day – his mouth was bleeding and his tongue was all dry, where he hadn't been cared for. I asked if he would like an ice lolly and he looked at me as if I was an angel, because he'd never even been offered one. I know it's hard in the hospital, but it doesn't take much.
>
> *Senior staff nurse 1*

Or very practical needs:

> To me, it's the simple things – the patient's care isn't finished until their environment is clean and tidy. If I were a relative and I came in and I saw tissues everywhere, towels lying everywhere, I would think, what have they done to my mum or dad? The patient also feels better if the area around them is good.
>
> *Head nurse*

> Someone who's gone home may need something, for instance a lift some-where and I might have a driver who could do that. There may be something about them which you can brief the volunteer on. I don't actually physically care for them, but it would be a bit weird if I didn't know them. It's being part of the whole community.
>
> *Volunteer coordinator*

> Money is a huge issue for people who are sick or dying. Some patients appear to be quite comfortable and then you discover that it's all a façade and they haven't got a bean! Sometimes I feel mighty irritated with the Benefits Agency or with charities who write to say they can't help a particular patient. It is hard work when someone's got no money. I know the charities that might help and write endless letters to them all.
>
> *Social worker*

Some may be thinking about how to improve future care:

> Food should be a sociable occasion. I like going to friends' houses and breaking the wine open – having a laugh and sharing the food. The patients take their medication in their bed, they poo and wee in their bed, they have the blood leaks and all the different things that happen when the system is breaking down – and then you bring them nice food and say 'here is your dinner'. It's important to get people away from their bed, away from the medical side.
>
> We want to have a separate dining area where people can sit with their families. When you walk into a restaurant, you look to see are the tables nice, are the glasses clean, do the waiters look presentable? And then you wonder does the food taste good? It is all about image and smell. We can put a nice linen cover on the table. One patient may be in a wheelchair and another with their Zimmer frame, and the family will have ordered lunch as well, so they are sitting there with their daughter, their wife, having lunch as if they are in a little restaurant somewhere. Yes, they are in the hospice, but they might feel that 'I am not in that room where I was in ter-rible pain last night'.
>
> *Chef*

Emotional help

There is also a need to address the emotional side:

> Somebody dying can be complicated. Sometimes, I take one relative away from
> the ward, speak to them and just get a picture of the family. My aim is to give
> them a chance to speak confidentially. Each person will be supporting the next
> person in that family, even if they don't realise it. By taking one individual out,
> it gives them space for their own thoughts and what's going on for them. Some
> families don't need any input – they are quite happy, very open. And some
> people, especially the older generation, have a stiff upper lip and just get on
> with it. There are a lot of very private people who don't want counselling.
>
> *Counsellor 1*

> I came from a very working class background with parents who were very
> much 'don't let anyone see that you're hurting – keep it all in'. A lot of our
> clients are working class people, so I can see where they're coming from.
> You look at some who are desperate to just let it all out – they have kept it
> all bottled up for so long. You begin to question the beliefs you were
> brought up with – why does it have to be that way?
>
> *Sister*

This can lead to unexpected revelations:

> As we get quite close to people, we get told things that they have never
> told anyone before – you have to listen and just be there for them. Sexual
> abuse has come up in men and women. They might be terminally ill and
> they will tell you that as a child, they were sexually abused by a member
> of the family – 'I have never told anybody this before, but I really need to
> get this off my chest before I go, do you mind if I talk to you?' and they let
> it all out. They are relieved, it is like a weight is off their shoulders – they
> might be in their seventies, eighties it doesn't matter what age they are.
>
> *Healthcare assistant 1*

> My conversation with them can lead to many, many things. They might
> talk about intimate things. They may look like a very devoted couple, but
> the wife will say 'well, he left me for five years in 1982'. All kinds of things
> open up – other wives, other families. We're a very small, intimate place.
> It's not a big busy hospital with people rushing in and out – the whole
> pace is much slower here.
>
> *Patient affairs officer*

Occasionally, there are problems in communication:

> We've had patients who don't speak any English. Then we have to rely a
> lot on their family or friends. We encourage them to stay if they can, and

if they can't, they will be on the end of the phone. We will have picture boards or we will have symbols, so we do try to do our best. We will also have people who understand English, but who can't vocalise or they're sign writers, so we will do whatever we can.

Senior staff nurse 2

I can think of a few cases where we haven't met someone's needs, for instance because their English is very limited. We obviously try to get an interpreter in, but sometimes it seems that their emotional distress is coming out more in physical symptoms that don't fit any particular pattern, such as all over body pain, not responding to any painkillers, emotional crying. You do feel out of your depth with that. If we were very concerned, we would get our social workers involved. The nurses are also better than us doctors with dealing with things, they have got to know the patient and the relatives much better than us, who sort of swan in and out.

Doctor 1

There was a gentleman recently, I can't remember whether he had had a stroke, but he just couldn't speak. You could see from his eyes that he had so much to say. If you can't speak, you feel trapped. Sometimes, we use a chalk board, but it is not like a conversation. I feel pretty useless when that happens. And some people are deaf. We had a chap who had a problem with his hearing and he was upset and I had to bellow at him. It doesn't sound very empathic, if you are bellowing 'how are you feeling?' You can't really do the work that is desperate to be done. And when you are working on the open ward, you are very aware that somebody else could be listening. You need to recognise that you can't always give the gold star service that you want to.

Counsellor 1

Spiritual support

Needs for spiritual support are also checked. This is done on admission and sometimes subsequently:

We always check what religion a patient is – that is fundamental. We will ask the patient if we are able to, or the family. A lot of people are Christian but not practising, but perhaps they would like somebody to come, so we check all that. For the Jewish and Muslim patients, it is really important for us to know what is going on, because when they die, everything needs to be done straightaway.

Staff nurse

When we have somebody admitted, we will always ask what their religion is and how orthodox they are or how strict they are to the codes. And whether they have their religious leader coming to visit them. Also how their relatives deal with their religion, because we may have Muslims, for example, who are very devout, but the younger generation haven't a clue what to do. We do quite a lot of exploring in order to prepare, so when the moment of death comes, there isn't huge confusion.

Senior staff nurse 2

Hospices have varying arrangements to accommodate such needs, both formal and informal:

One day a week, we have a service in the prayer room. On two other days, the chaplain will arrive and just talk to people. We have one chaplain who is on duty for the week, who will endeavour to come in every day and meet the patients and relatives and build up any relationships that patients might want. It's amazing what will come out of a conversation. They don't always talk about God, but they see a person who they feel can listen to them and won't judge them. That's the biggest thing people are fearful of – being judged. It's really a fear of God's judgement. I always say 'it's not for me to judge you – by judging you, I would be judging myself and that's inappropriate'.

Chaplain 2

Patients are always very happy to talk. I always start by asking fairly neutral questions that don't disturb them – where they live, where they come from. Then I ask if there's something I can do for them in particular. Patients don't tend to discuss what will happen when they die and I would never say 'you've got to prepare yourself'. They know perfectly well what's going to happen. If patients have had a good relationship with their own parish priest, they will expect me to continue that relationship as someone who is helping them at a very special time.

Chaplain 1

Chaplains feel that they are there to be available and to listen, but are careful not to press themselves on patients:

I see a chaplain's role as sort of 'loitering with intent'. I go to the nurses' station to say that I'm here and, if it's a quiet time, then usually the senior nurse will go through the people who are in beds and maybe steer me in a particular direction. If they're busy, I go onto the wards and introduce myself. I say that I'm there on behalf of the chaplaincy team and, judging on their reactions, how well or unwell a person is feeling on that day, I might be invited to stay. It might just be a conversation, it just depends. Or it might just be me sitting a little while, with no conversation.

Sometimes people want nothing from me, because they're very angry with God for whatever reason – and I'm God's representative. I've never been rejected directly, except in the mildest form. It's body language when families don't particularly want a chaplain. Sometimes, they're waiting for relatives and they just want company. Or they want somebody to share something, someone who they know is not there for any other purpose but to be alongside. On some occasions, it feels a bit like a confessional and that's absolutely safe. It's a space in which they can offload regret. And a place of prayer if that's their wish.

Chaplain 3

Indeed, they may well talk to people with other belief systems:

We're not here to convert people to Christianity. We're here to support them the best way we can with their spiritual fears and aspirations. Some ministers see their job to be to convert people before they die. That's not what we're here for. We will talk to a patient if they want us to talk to them. It's the patient's autonomy that matters. They have the right to ask me to leave them alone.

Chaplain 2

I embrace people of other faiths. Some people have a spirituality that is very different to mine. It may not be religious beliefs, but a working out of who they are and why they're here. I've not actually engaged with anybody for whom the notion of God was non-existent, but there are those who want a closer relationship with God, to feel encouraged by faith and life beyond. If somebody wants to ask questions about their faith, I'm on hand to assist that, but initially I'm just alongside them.

I had an interesting experience with a woman who professed to be a witch and a pagan. She shunned counselling services, but was willing to have a dialogue with a representative from the chaplaincy. I found her difficult, because I was being invited to share in some kind of ritual of a pagan nature. The question in my mind was 'how far do I engage with this person – when is it OK to say no, I'd prefer not to?' I said that I would need some time to think about it and I think we never re-visited it.

Chaplain 3

Discussions about returning home

During a stay in a hospice, there may be discussions of whether patients would like to go back home for a period and any difficulties this might entail:

It is different for different people. At the moment, we have one lady who has been here for symptom control and really wants to go home. I will go through the things that have to be done, like the medicine, and will ask if she needs help with anything at home. I have another lady going home alone and that is always a danger point. We will have a case conference and we will invite the district nurses, the palliative care team, the doctors, myself, the patient and the family to sit down together and talk about concerns that may arise. She had a personal safety device, but because of a physical problem, she can't activate it. She had had two falls previously at home, so it is a matter of getting someone to make it possible for her to just kick the bathroom skirting board and get help.

Occasionally, I will question something. We have got a gentleman at the moment and the doctor has him well under control medically, the nurses say they have done all they can for him, but I am not sure he can do the stairs and his bed is upstairs. I want a physiotherapist's assessment. The doctors are good – if I say I am concerned about safety issues, they will give me a bit longer. We all do it together, but the final say would be with the doctors or the nurses.

Discharge nurse 1

And there may be a discussion about where they want to die:

One question we ask is where do they want to die – at home or here in the hospice? Most people want to die at home, so we support that. I've just been in touch with social services to say I've got a chap who is going to be looking at going home – I want somebody going in four times to help with personal care for himself and the preparation of meals, a bit of shopping, laundry, cleaning the house and so forth. Social services are quite happy with that. We only need a district nurse to go in to do the medication. We need to sort out a line that you wear round your neck and it's registered with a call centre day and night, for people living alone where there's an emergency. You obviously have to ask the patient, but most of them want to go home.

Discharge nurse 2

I encourage people to die at home – home is a nicer environment, it's their own environment. What right do I have to take them from that to die in the hospice, when all the services and everything could be put into the home? But I always give them options. The decision about where a patient should die is done with discretion with the patient or family member. Some patients just don't want to face it and you have to respect their choice. I had one guy who died just recently and he'd walk out the room if I even broached the subject of the future. In the end, he died at home – his wife wanted him at home and even when he was becoming weaker, he'd say 'I'm fine, I'm fine, I'm good'. The week before he died, I'd seen him at home and he looked straight in my face and I think he knew. I said 'I'll come back and see you in a couple of days' and he said 'yes, that will be great'. I think he was saying goodbye in his own way.

Community nurse

Most people want to die in their own home, although only 25–30% of people manage it. And there are a significant number who would like to die in a hospice – there are advantages to each. There are plenty of people who don't have family or a family who are capable of managing – obviously, the hospice is the ideal situation for them. Also, some complications and symptoms around dying need ongoing specialist support in order to keep a person comfortable – and there, the hospice is an ideal setting.

Consultant

The needs of relatives and friends

Equally, a lot of work revolves around a patient's family or close friends, who may be around for long periods of time:

Relatives can be here 24/7. I welcome that. These people have got a very limited time left with their loved ones and they should be able to be with the person. We've not got the right to take time away from them. I've seen that with both my parents. Some staff say that it makes their job harder – they tend to be people that haven't lost someone.

Sister

Again, efforts are made to assess their particular needs and to respond to them:

Often, you will find that you are much more involved with one family compared to another. It is like anything in life, you meet people that you gel with. Some people are also more needy and you have to sort of weigh up – do they want me to back off? Do they want me to come and sit with them? I take things very slowly. We are here for 13 hours, so they may say hello and turn their back and shut the door, that's fine, but a couple of hours later, they may meet me in the corridor and stop me. You almost have a sixth sense for the ones that need somebody to just sit and be there.

Healthcare assistant 1

When I first came here, families used to go out and get a sandwich. I thought why are we taking people away, when the patient could die and they have missed that moment. That one moment – they may have missed it! So we decided to supply food for sale. And the money we make gets ploughed back into the hospice, to help fund all the fresh vegetables and meat.

Chef

I am here to support patients and anybody affected by a patient's illness. It doesn't have to be family – it can be friends, neighbours. I go down onto the wards and let myself be known to people. I take it very gently at first, because people tend to think they must have something very wrong if they need to see a counsellor. I just tell them who I am and say 'I am here for each of you'. I try to get eye contact with several people in the room, so I am not directing this to just one person. Sometimes they will catch me in the corridor and say 'actually, I would like some time, but I didn't want Mum to know'. Once people talk, the floodgates open.

Counsellor 1

Sometimes, there is a need for a small amount of reciprocation, to build up rapport:

They're interested just a little bit about you, but you can't give too much information. I would say I live nearby, I've got a little niece – because if you're always probing them, it's a bit one-sided. I give them a little bit about my life, just to give them some feedback and build up their trust. I don't tell them anything about how I am feeling.

Community nurse

Occasionally, staff can find themselves caught up in a complex web of relationships:

Families can disagree on the management of a patient's disease – some wanting more aggressive treatment, which is really not appropriate. That's not uncommon. You have to moderate between family members, bringing them together from different standpoints. Mostly it is achievable, if you're prepared to chip away at it.

Consultant

There is always dynamics in families. We see somebody who is unwell – we don't know what they were like when they were well. We don't know what sort of parent they were – or sister or brother. If we have a patient who has six children and none of them visit, there is a reason for that – and that's between them. I never, ever question that, because none of us know what's gone on in their lives. If they want to tell us why, that's up to them.

If a patient is here for a while, they might open up and say they have children who they haven't seen for years. I might ask whether they want to contact them, but mostly they will say no. You have to respect their wishes. Some people may want this happy little package, where it has all come together at the end and they have all said what they should have said, but that doesn't happen in real life. What gets said doesn't get erased sometimes. And that's up to them – our business is caring for the person who is dying.

When relatives come into the building, they have to go to the reception, say who they are and who they are visiting. The receptionist phones the nurse's office and they have to say if the patient's visitor is allowed down. Sometimes they might not feel up to visitors, but you also get situations where there are members of their family who they don't want to see. We have to tell the visitor 'actually, we can't let you come in'. That's OK, because I am there for the protection of the patient. If it is going to cause distress that somebody has turned up out of the blue, I am not there to judge. It doesn't happen very often.

Healthcare assistant 1

We see a person and that may not be the person the family know. We had one patient who was a very nice man until it came to discharge, then the family wouldn't have him back. He had serially abused his daughter and his granddaughter and they'd had a rest from him and they just couldn't go back to it – but to us he was a lovely man.

Head nurse

Family members may also become involved in day centre activities:

I say to people who attend the centre that this is your space, your place to come for whatever reason, your sanctuary. If you find that you'd like to show it to family or friends, they can come as guests for lunch, which kind of normalises it. If someone says to me that they'd really like me to meet their family member, partner, friend, then we'd set up a proper meeting. Very often we'll get to know the family well, which is very nice if people end up going into the hospice. Then we know the family dynamic and we can continue to play a part, because the family may come to talk through things with me or other staff at the centre about what's happening for them. This can feel supportive and safe.

Some family members can be very anxious about losing their role as the major source of support. So they can be very suspect of us and of the relationship that we're going to create. They come in saying 'I know what my mother wants' and will insist on the need to be here. We work with that very gently, very slowly, we tell them we're going to take really good care of the person. We recognise that the relationship that they have is very special. And generally, if they know that they can come and visit, gradually the anxieties ease off. We're always asking the patient's permission— 'is it OK with you if your daughter comes to visit with us from time to time?' 'Is it OK if we talk with her about how things are going for you?' I use OK or all right a lot in conversations, asking permission from the patient 'can we do this? Is this all right?'

Day centre manager

Children

It is not uncommon for patients to have young children or grandchildren who visit the hospice:

We get lots of children visiting people at the hospice. We have a very well worked out programme of support that includes a children's room with toys to try to make children feel welcome. The social workers would make a point of trying to be involved with families as much as possible, where there are young children involved – whether they're grandchildren or children, and would hope to work with those families offering as much or as little support as those families want.

Social worker

It hurts when you go in and see them. You know that you can't change this event and it's going to have a big impact on their life. You see them playing and you think, God, they shouldn't have to experience this. It always chokes me up to see them – they end up growing up without their parent, maybe without really knowing them.

Head of hospice 1

And efforts may be made to help the children or parents:

There was one lady who had teenage daughters and she didn't want them to have any counselling. She said that they know what's going on, they're fine, she'd spoken to them about it, which she had. But we knew how much it would help them. Children need to know what's going on. We've seen before how upsetting it can be if you don't allow teenagers to express what they're feeling. Some people think counselling means they're going to be psychoanalysed. I tend to use the term 'family worker' now.

We lost another woman who had two young daughters and she didn't want counselling either. We managed to get her to write the girls a letter each. She didn't exactly put in it what I would have done – I probably would have said that I'm really proud of them and I love them, but she was more saying 'make sure you do this and make sure you do that'. But at least she got it done.

Senior staff nurse 1

CHAPTER 4

Working with dying people

Although people who work in hospices are not all dealing with an actual death every day, it is a common part of their day-to-day work. This chapter explores some of the issues involved in attending to the needs of dying people and their families.

Helping people to come to terms with dying

The process of dying is not always straightforward. People can have days when they are slowly deteriorating as well as days when they feel better. Nurses and others can spend a lot of time helping people to come to terms with their situation:

> Patients often ask us if they are dying. I tend to ask 'how do you feel? What do you think is happening?' Often, they will say that they feel weaker and I would agree with them. In most cases, patients do know – they recognise that they are getting weaker, that they are dying, but sometimes they just want to ask.
>
> *Senior staff nurse 3*

> A lot of it is just answering questions. Sometimes they'll ask if they're going to die. I usually say something like 'well, obviously that's going to happen to all of us, but what is the main concern for you?' And then they talk about it a bit more. I don't talk about death and dying if they don't bring it up. Some people don't want to talk about it. They know and I know they know – and that's the way they want to deal with it.
>
> *Community nurse*

> I wonder if it isn't an arrogance to feel we do anything. In the end, people do it themselves. They draw on their own inner resources. But there is a role to play. You are alongside someone – you are here with them. You can reassure them that someone will be there holding their hand, that we won't leave them or we'll help them sort out something they're very worried about.
>
> *Social worker*

Being alert to these questions is seen as important:

> What all nurses need to know is if they're asked a question and they can't answer it or don't want to answer it, they must get somebody who *will*

answer it straightaway – because that patient may never find the courage to ask that question again. Some nurses find it very difficult to impart bad news – if someone asks 'am I dying?' They will say 'no, of course you're not'. They don't want to take hope away. We send them on courses, but they still find it very difficult.

Head nurse

Some patients may be very frightened:

A lot of people just want to be blotted out – they can't cope with thinking about dying. They will say they're in pain, so you give them lots of drugs and then they sleep all the time. It always distresses me. I can understand younger doctors having difficulties, as I did, in really being open and honest and saying 'look, I think you want these drugs so you don't have to think about what's happening to you, rather than trying to find ways of coping with it'.

Most patients are afraid of dying, whether or not they're saying it, there is a fear. It's just the unknown. They've never been this route before and what's going to happen? How is it going to happen? Where am I going? The fear of leaving people – find me anyone who isn't really apprehensive about that! I'm apprehensive, myself.

Consultant

If somebody said to me 'I'm dying, I'm really frightened', I would explore with them what their fear is. And having done that so many times, their fear is the journey to death. Maybe one person in fifty will say it's the death itself. Mostly it's that journey, because they're not sure what it's going to be like. Both the pain they might suffer and how it will be at that last minute for them.

I try to get a real feel about whether they want to talk. I made mistakes early on. I can remember talking to one man about death and dying and that's not where he wanted to go. I was not picking up the signals. It was almost like my mission, I thought this was what I was employed to do. That was really the worst error I've made and it was certainly a wake-up call.

Counsellor 2

There can be particular problems with people who do not speak English:

In most cases, there would be somebody we can communicate with. There was one patient whose husband didn't speak any English – she was too unwell to translate and we needed to get an interpreter to help us to explain things. It was difficult, because usually you would be updating and explaining as the day goes along, but it was only the one chance to get all the important things over. Luckily, that does not happen very often.

Senior staff nurse 3

Of course, chaplains or other religious leaders may be brought in at this stage:

> We call the chaplain for them, if they ask. If a person is close to dying, we
> would ask the family or sometimes the family will approach us. You get to
> know the families who are deeply religious. I've been nursing so long, it's
> like a seventh sense.
>
> *Senior staff nurse 1*

> I've often found it's enough just to be with people. You don't actually have
> to give words of consolation, which can perhaps sound artificial, but just
> be with them. Often, they start talking and you respond. People don't
> really want to think of death. We cling to life as long as possible. We talk
> about eternal life and physical death is not the end of all, that the spirit
> lives on. The Last Rites used to be called extreme unction and people used
> to be fearful. The Church has changed the name to the Anointing of the
> Sick to help people who are seriously ill – it doesn't have a sense of final-
> ity. You can repeat the Anointing as often as you feel it helps. Eventually,
> it does become the Last Rites or the Last Anointing.
>
> The Anointing is spiritual, but it's also emotional and psychological. It
> gives people peace, they're being prepared for death, the Church itself is
> helping them and blessing them. We believe that it is one of the sacra-
> ments and it does have the effect of easing a person's mind and heart.
>
> *Chaplain 1*

Dying people continue to have a variety of needs and staff do their best to cater for
them:

> I have been working with a lady who wanted to write letters to her grand-
> children. I had a sense of urgency that it needed to be done today, because
> she is not well. She wanted to leave it till tomorrow, so it was on my agenda
> to get it done today. I just said to her 'why don't we just talk about what
> you want to get done?' I spent quite a long time, just sitting in her room
> and letting her doze – and then she talked. Gradually, stuff started to
> come out, so I just said 'shall we just make some pointers on a bit of paper,
> just as you are telling me?' I spent about an hour and a half with her and
> we got these letters written.
>
> *Counsellor 1*

> People need time at the end. We all keep secrets when we're alive – if you
> knew the day you are going to die, you would undo all the bad things you
> have done. If we get hit by a car, we don't have that choice. But if you have
> a patient who comes in and doesn't eat, they just go into a sleep mode, they
> are never going to deal with issues that their family might want to talk
> about. Maybe they had a fight a year ago – people do keep little petty
> thoughts in their head. So if we feed them and get their energy levels up,

they can actually communicate more. They can have quality time with each other, they might bring up the subject 'oh, remember last year, I fought with you and I'm really sorry' – it affects the quality of dying. Because when people have cleaned the slate, they die happier – or as happy as you can die.

No one has ever showed me the brochure of the other side, but I am not keen on it myself. They say the last sense to go is your hearing, so you can maybe hear your family talking about you, but you cannot communicate back to them. So through feeding them, you have got that bit of strength and you can have that little conversation you should have had a year ago.

Chef

Relatives may also need attention:

Some relatives may have fears around the death and what it's going to be like – are they going to be in pain? Will they be vomiting? Is it something I can physically and mentally cope with? If you've never seen anybody die before, 'how will I know?' Then they have the dilemma about whether they should have the children here or not or who should be present. What if they miss it? That's a big issue.

Head of hospice 1

This is also a time for dealing with various practical matters:

We have a legal responsibility for both Jewish and Muslim patients to be seen by a doctor on a Friday evening, because if they die on the Sabbath, they have to be buried within 24 hours. I can ring the doctor on a Friday evening and all he has to do is pop his head round the door and say 'doctor here, are you OK? Just checking'. It's a formality, but it is a very important thing that the doctor gets to see them, because if they've not been seen, we can't do a death certificate.

Discharge nurse 2

I'm quite passionate about organ donation. I like to make patients aware that even though they've got cancer, they can still donate corneas and things like that. So if I know a patient's got a donor card, I get a little piece written into the folder to allow people to make that decision if they want.

Senior staff nurse 1

It's horrible to be asking somebody who's only got a few days to live to sign their will. There was a patient with motor neurone disease who wanted to change his will and leave it all to his ex-wife. We asked the family to leave and the two of us sat down – it took ages because his speech was very slow. I needed to make sure that I was 100% happy that what he was doing was the right thing and that nobody was putting him under pressure – that what he'd signed was what he wanted.

Head of hospice 1

Very occasionally, patients or families will ask about opportunities to end it all:

A couple of people at home have wanted to go to Switzerland because that's where they do euthanasia. I've said it's illegal here, so I can't help you, but they're asking me for information and I say 'well, why do you feel the need to end it?' And then they come out with the fact that they're going to be in a lot of pain, they're alone, things like that. So I discuss what we can put in place to ensure that that doesn't happen.

Community nurse

We've started to have these questions – people ask us 'can you not give them something?' I say it's illegal, it's against the law and we just cannot. You sympathise with them and you say let's try and work out why you want it. Is the pain not sorted out? Are the symptoms not sorted? If they're comfortable, then they should be able to enjoy the last period of their life. Sometimes it's the family who can't cope with the situation.

Head of hospice 1

I'm looking after a woman with advanced motor neurone disease – she's pretty well paralysed, using a ventilator – and we had a long talk about assisted suicide, because it's been in the news. She was very eloquent, saying 'I don't think I would want that, but I might – and who are you to say what I feel I need for myself?' I said 'you're absolutely right'. The general palliative care community is very against it, but I just feel unless you're in that position, how can you possibly know? I have known a very small number of patients who would have finished themselves off, but it's been very, very small. So it's not a major issue.

Consultant

Returning home to die

Arrangements may be made for people who want to die at home:

If someone wants to die at home, if it's conceivably possible, we'll get them home. Obviously, if their families feel they can't cope or there's nobody at home, it's very difficult. We've had a couple of patients who wanted to go home to die and their families felt that they couldn't cope. Eventually, the doctors managed to persuade the patients that they'd be much better looked after here. It can be hard at home, unless you have somebody who doesn't have many symptoms and is just going to slip away nice and peacefully.

Senior staff nurse 1

If a patient wants to die at home, I would go straight to the family. If the patient is conscious and able to speak, I would obviously include them, but very often the mother, say, is unconscious and the family have said they want her back home, it is where she wants to be. In that case, I will immediately draw up paperwork and notify the district nurses. And I will alert the palliative care team in the community, because they have to have medicines readily available for injection, draw up syringe driver charts, arrange ambulances. In my experience, everybody is absolutely fantastic.

I have only had one situation where the palliative care team were very reluctant, saying they were too short staffed to be able to visit. It was a Friday and it would have been the weekend, but the family were adamant and, in truth, it wasn't rocket science, it was just letting somebody die. It went ahead and it was a comfortable death. The transport people are absolutely fantastic. They can be so busy, but I have always found that they will do it. It seems to bring out the best in people.

Discharge nurse 1

And sometimes, a person will want to return to their home country. If left too late, this can be very difficult:

I got involved with a lady from the Philippines, who was only in her early forties. We knew that she was going to die, but by the time she agreed it was the time, she wasn't well enough to travel. They wouldn't allow her to get on the plane. We raised funds to bring her husband over, but when he arrived he spoke no English and could speak only a rare dialect, so we had to find somebody who could interpret. He wanted to take her back to the Philippines to see the children, but that required a private ambulance which turned out to cost £100,000. He was quite angry – I couldn't understand what he was saying, but you could tell by his whole body language. I felt disappointed I couldn't get her back to see her children, because if it was my mum, how would I cope with the fact that she went away for a number of years and then died and I never saw her again?

Head of hospice 1

Recognising the terminal phase

Experienced nurses and doctors tend to know when the end is in sight, although it is never wholly predictable. Initially, there can be a kind of restlessness:

You recognise the signs that someone's now in a terminal phase. The patient's behaviour changes, they're not comfortable. It's not necessarily any pain or discomfort, but generally just not knowing what they want. The patient also gets weaker.

Senior staff nurse 3

One of the signs is that people become restless. They suddenly want to get out of bed, they want to go home and they just become very anxious. We call that 'terminal restlessness'. It is not something you can explain, because it is not actually where they should be at. Just the signs of somebody deteriorating – colour changes, perhaps a moist chest so you can hear them, a bit of confusion perhaps, disorientation and then just a decline into becoming unresponsive at some point.

Staff nurse

Family are informed and even more attention is paid to the patient's needs:

Most of the time, we have some idea of how close the person is to dying, so that we can let the family know. We would make sure that we would be around. I always say to the family 'I am here, you might see me at the door, I might come to the bed. I am not going to invade your privacy, but if I feel things are getting nearer the time, I will tell you'. And they are very grateful for that. I try to keep in the background, but I let them know I am there.

Healthcare assistant 1

We tend to recognise things quite early, that things are changing, different drugs are required. Sometimes it's an internal pain that medicines can't fix. I try to talk to them about that and to family members about saying it's OK to let go. That that's quite important. I just say that when their time is coming, it's OK and they can actually let go. Some worry about the relatives – I say that I think they will be all right, they just want to know that you're OK.

Community nurse

But death remains somewhat unpredictable, so this can be a difficult time for everyone:

Sometimes it really is not predictable. We will have someone who looks like they are going to die and then they just don't. It is a very hard call to make and we say so. We say to families this may not be it, but do you want to be here if we think it is? Then they make a choice as to whether they're going to come in.

It is really difficult for families when you call them in because somebody has deteriorated – and then they rally. Then they deteriorate and you call them in again and tell them that you think this might be it – and then it is not. It's one of the hardest things here. But generally people can be prepared. Some patients go more quickly than expected and then we have to deal with that as well, because families get here too late.

Staff nurse

The actual death

As death approaches, patients generally seem to go very quiet:

> Mostly you know when someone is about to die. People are quite drowsy
> and you will notice changes in their breathing. Sometimes people will say
> the name of their mother or sister or somebody who has died in the past.
> That's quite a good indication that something's happening which we can't
> see. Sometimes, there's a change in their appearance. They may seem
> more peaceful.
>
> *Senior staff nurse 2*

> When someone's approaching death, what you notice is a distinctive
> smell, a bit like the air spray that smells like vanilla. That's the first thing
> you notice if you go near a patient who's near to death. You can never
> gauge how soon. Sometimes, you can just turn your back and someone
> will go. You have just gone out the room to get something and you come
> back and he has gone.
>
> *Nurse 1*

Hospice staff generally do everything they can to enable a death to go smoothly. This
means respecting what the patient and families want:

> A lot of people whisper or talk very quietly, when someone is dying. I
> always encourage them to carry on talking, because the patient can still
> hear – hearing is the last thing to go. We also encourage them to bring in
> their favourite music, for instance Irish music for an Irish girl, and we will
> play it continuously. It is mostly cheerful – it is very rare to get someone
> who will have morbid music. If your family are all there and it makes it
> happy, a person passes away just nicely, I would treat that as a good death.
>
> *Nurse 1*

> There was one Muslim man who had already had their religious leader,
> and it was at that terminal stage where the patient is unresponsive and all
> the family is there. I had said 'I don't know your religion, is there anything
> I can do?' They asked if we could turn the bed. Physically turn it – the
> head has to go to the east and the cleric recites prayers until the death. I
> felt I'd done what the family had wanted.
>
> *Nurse 2*

There may be issues about who is present:

> If somebody is dying, about half the time we're with them. Sometimes we
> can't be there at the moment of death and a relative will be with them, but
> we'll be in and out quite a few times. Some relatives actually don't want
> you there – things are going OK and they're comfortable with how things

are. They will press the buzzer when the breathing has changed – maybe there's one or two breaths left and they call you back for that.

Senior staff nurse 2

We ask the family if they want us to stay. Almost invariably, we will be in the room, even if we are not right at the bed. You can see by the anxiety in the room whether or not you need to be there. Death is not glamorous – somebody might be pouring fluid all over the place, so you're trying to manage that, trying to be discreet around suctioning that person. Also, it can be an issue where families are definitely not accepting the death and not letting that person go.

Staff nurse

Families may have particular needs at the point of death:

Families are often frightened at the moment of death because they might not have experienced a death before. It is also a bit scary for me, even though I have done it for a long time. Sometimes you think that somebody has passed away and there can be this huge gap, minutes, and then they take another gasp – that's quite upsetting for the people there. So we are there, discreetly – we sort of step back, but we watch for the rhythm and we make sure that we let them know that they have passed away.

Healthcare assistant 1

If patients have no family, staff will do their best to be with them:

We have patients who have nobody – no relatives, no friends, nothing – it's horrendous. Or sometimes relatives can't get here in time. To the utmost of our ability, we will make sure that one of us is with them. No matter what happens in your life, no one should be dying on their own. If someone is waiting for a relative to arrive, we reassure them and say they are on the way. We had a woman recently who didn't have anyone apart from her brother in Africa and we just kept saying 'he's coming, just sleep until he gets here'.

Senior staff nurse 4

Sometimes, nurses are reluctant to leave, even if it is at the end of a shift:

It's hard, very hard, to leave someone who is dying. If you've spent all day with somebody and you're very close to the relatives, you want to be there. You want to be the one consoling the relatives, making sure that they are fine up until the end. Even though I know they're going to be fine, because my colleagues are more than capable to continue that for me. But you do build up attachment and it's stupid for anyone to say that we don't or we shouldn't. We are human beings – not robots.

Senior staff nurse 4

It is thought that people's beliefs can affect a death:

> Some people are able to let go. I have learned from working here, a lot of what happens can be what's happened in their life. Very often, if people have a strong faith, they accept death a lot easier than somebody who is agnostic or an atheist. Fear comes into it – fear of the unknown, fear of suffering pain. And the same with the families.
>
> *Healthcare assistant 1*

> We've nursed people of all religions. It's easier where people believe in life after death. Hindu patients who think they're coming back – being rein-carnated – can be more fearful in terms of whether or not they've achieved something, because there's a whole thing on achieving greater levels. They might be coming back as a lower thing, so there's a lot of fear around death. It's different for Muslims. Life is complete for them, death is a completion and they accept that it's over.
>
> *Staff nurse*

A doctor or chaplain may be nearby, but will not necessarily be present at the moment of death:

> I'm not often with patients when they die. I might be called because the relatives believe the person is at the end – and then it might happen whilst I'm there. But more often than not, I would share with the family and then prayers and the person would perhaps be only a few hours away from death.
>
> *Chaplain 3*

> There are a few times when I've actually been there – if I notice a patient is dying, I stay. But if I'm not there, sometimes the relatives call me, because they want a doctor to be there to say whether it has happened. I'll go.
>
> *Doctor 2*

Some deaths are seen primarily as a relief:

> Some patients after they've died, look so peaceful – and you think all that pain has gone. There was a lady we had here who I knew before. She had a cancer and then she got cancer somewhere else and then cancer some-where else and you think how much more can somebody take? So when she died, I was so relieved for her, because she suffered beyond belief. She never complained and you think 'you poor little love'. So sometimes it's a happy release.
>
> *Healthcare assistant 2*

The occasional death is difficult:

> We had a woman who had been in and out a few times, an elderly woman, with a lovely sense of humour. She had gone to the toilet one night and locked the toilet door. We noticed she wasn't in her bed for quite a long time – myself and another nurse had to find a way to open the door and found her dead. That upset us. We expect people to die peacefully and comfortably in their beds, but life isn't like that. People do die suddenly in all sorts of places.
>
> *Senior staff nurse 2*

> We had an Afro-Caribbean woman, who was only in her mid-forties. Her son and daughter were not very supportive. When she was admitted, it became obvious that she was absolutely terrified of dying. She had joined a fundamentalist evangelical church and they came and prayed around her bed every day, but it didn't seem to give her any peace. It got to a point where she couldn't sleep, because she was so frightened that she'd die when she went to sleep. Eventually, her mother arrived from the Caribbean – she saw her mother and lay down on her bed. She was so exhausted that she went to sleep and died. I've never forgotten her tormented face.
>
> *Social worker*

But some deaths are remembered as being particularly special:

> We had a man who was Buddhist who died the other week – his brothers asked me what we had for Buddhists. I said we didn't really have anything, but anyone was more than welcome to come in. Because we knew he was deteriorating, they managed to get Buddhist monks who were all chanting and chiming as he was dying. It was beautiful, really lovely.
>
> *Senior staff nurse 4*

> I was on night duty recently and, coming to the end of my break, I was sitting in the prayer room. A girl came in whose mother was dying. She said she didn't know if there was a God, but she was afraid she wouldn't see her mother again and she felt very alone. We talked a bit about the Ascension and about when our Lord said 'there are many rooms in my Father's house'. We were having a prayer between ourselves at the end and one of my colleagues came in and said to her 'you need to go back to your mum'. Her breathing had changed and she was dying. The daughter and a friend started singing a hymn. And the mother died with this going on around her. I thought that was beautiful, absolutely beautiful. The daughter was really upset, but she'd done what she wanted to do with her mum. She'd been there for her.
>
> *Senior staff nurse 2*

There was one priest who died here and I have never seen anything like it. He was completely at peace. Physically, he was OK, but it was very much like the curtains are drawn and there is a light there and I am so looking forward to meeting my Maker. That was pretty amazing, you rarely see that.

Doctor 1

CHAPTER 5

After a death

Once a patient dies, there are a range of tasks to be done, both immediately and in the longer term. A hospice's relationship with families does not end with the death, but may continue for some time.

Giving time to families

At the point of death, the first requirement is to enable families to have time with the person who died:

> Once the death happens, I say 'I am going to leave the room, I am just going to be outside if you need me, but spend some time.' After about half an hour or so, we will go in and say 'come and have a cup of tea, we are going to make them comfortable'. That may sound a funny word when somebody has died, but we would go in then and make the person more presentable. Their mouth might be wide open, they may have died in a position where they are all crumpled up in the bed.
>
> We lay them out, we don't wash them then, but maybe wipe their face, brush their hair, maybe bring some flowers into the room, and take out any medical equipment. It's a bit of a rush. We empty the room except for all their personal things, maybe a pair of glasses, their flowers, things that the family know belong to the person. And then we bring the family back down and ask if they would like to see them. They look like they are sleeping – tidy and nice. The suction machine is not there anymore, the oxygen has gone. And we say to them 'spend some time' – they can stay for half an hour or stay for hours.
>
> *Healthcare assistant 1*

Families have very differing needs:

> All relatives are different. Some take it well – they will have their tears and say their goodbyes. But some are very distraught. You just need to be with them. You put your arm round them, give them a hug or put your hand on them. Or if the person has died and they're hugging that person, you just stand back and allow them to be, because that's their moment. You can't take that away. Obviously, there will come a point, maybe after a few hours, where you would try to encourage them that now is the time to leave. That

doesn't happen very often, surprisingly. Most people find the 'right' time to leave the deceased person.

Senior staff nurse 2

I didn't know what to say to families when I first worked here, but I've learned how to approach them. They don't need sympathy, they don't need you hugging and kissing them, they just really need practical help. They're grieving anyway – just say 'how can I help you? What do you need?'

Senior staff nurse 1

I have been present at some deaths. You have to be really careful, because they may try to get you to state that maybe the person has gone to heaven. You can't do that. So when somebody dies, it's really about putting the hand out – just being there, so they're not by themselves. Even small things like tissues, a cup of tea, just saying, 'how are you feeling about things now?' Very mundane things.

Counsellor 2

Some are frightened of being with a dead body:

Families can be really stressed. I will ask if they are OK, because some people are scared stiff to be left on their own with someone who's passed away. If they don't want to go on their own, we will go in with them. If they still don't want to go in, we will respect their views – they have got the right to say no. Sometimes it is better to see the person when they were alive than to see them when they have died, when they are a bit paler. Remembering how you last saw them alive is the best memory you can have.

Nurse 1

People do find it difficult to be with dead bodies and touching people. It's something about our culture – people should be looking at death and dying the whole of their lives, so it becomes part and parcel of what happens in life. There's a lot of people who just won't talk about it, even at the very end.

Counsellor 2

Occasionally, relatives find it difficult to let go:

After they have seen the person, we explain that they will be able to see them tomorrow, but maybe it is time they went home and got some rest. And they are normally very good at saying yes, they will go. But I have experienced people who have literally hung onto the bed and just refused, they have been so distraught and they just cried and cried. You have to give them time – eventually they cry it out. It's heartbreaking to see that.

Healthcare assistant 1

Preparing the body

The next step is for the body to be washed and prepared:

What happens after a death depends on the culture. We would be guided by the family and what they want us to do. In most cases, they would wish us to wash the patient. Some people want to have family there when we're doing that, but some don't – it's their choice. Obviously, we would straighten them up and make sure that they're laying properly. We always explain that to the family. For a Jewish patient, they would get their own people to do the washing – they have a protocol about how they do it.

Senior staff nurse 3

I would always ask the family if there is anything I can or I can't do – that is just common sense and courtesy. When one Muslim man died, the daughters came out and I said I was sorry and asked what I could or could not do, as I did not want to offend their religion. I explained that we would take the catheter out and give him a wash down. The daughter said that was fine, provided it's men that do it.

Nurse 2

Nurses continue to think of the patient as a person, not as a body:

We wash them and put a gown on and wrap them up in a sheet and then the porters come and take them away. Even though someone has passed away, you are still talking to them, to ease your own mind. We always talk to the patient – they are still our patient until they leave. So while washing them, we will say 'come on, just roll towards me' and we will still say 'sorry' if we drop our grasp for a second, 'oh, sorry about that'. We also say 'you have had your family, now you are at rest, you are free from pain, have a nice sleep now', just like that. It is just very comforting to say all these things.

Nurse 1

Most people working in a hospice for any period of time will have had the opportunity to get used to handling a dead body, but for new people it can be difficult:

When new nurses are not used to dealing with death, that can be hard. That happened to me not so long ago. I didn't know this nurse had never worked with death. A patient passed away and I said I needed a hand to wash them – and she just froze on the spot. I said 'you roll the person and

I will do the washing' and she didn't move. She had gone white – I asked if she had ever worked with someone who has passed away and she hadn't. I sat her down and got her a cup of tea and found another nurse to help me. I felt sorry for her. Some people get very frightened and you have to comfort them.

Nurse 1

If it is expected that relatives will be coming later, the body may be moved to a special room for the purpose:

When somebody dies, the bed is wheeled into what we call the family room. We can control the temperature in there – we can take it down like a fridge for practicality. We always ask relatives if there is anybody else coming to visit and if someone is coming from a distance, we keep the body in that room. The nurses are very good at making a body look nice, positioning the hands, rosary beads, flowers between the fingers. Some relatives have commented that's how they're going to remember their mum – 'she looked really nice and peaceful'.

The sofa in the family room is put in front of the nurses' station. So if anyone comes in to the hospice in the morning and the sofa is there, it means somebody has died and there's somebody in the room.

Nurse 2

A special room is particularly important where families are from a culture which involves wailing, as this can be disturbing for other patients:

We had a Muslim gentleman some weeks ago and the family warned us that there would be lots of chanting. So we put the patient in a room that we knew wouldn't affect the rest of the building and we shut the two doors – the women fell on the floor, they wailed, they banged their chests, the men were chanting. If it had gone on for ages, we would have had to ask them to stop, but they respected the fact that there were other patients here.

Healthcare assistant 1

One thing we can find difficult is where some cultures practise wailing. Part of that is the impact it may have on other patients. We have a viewing room at the back of the hospice. If we know a family where wailing is likely to happen, we try to get the patient round there as quickly as possible, so that if it does occur, it will occur there. If it does upset the patients, then we would just explain it's nothing to be afraid of, it is a cultural thing.

Head nurse

For those whose religion requires immediate burial, attention must also be given to the paperwork:

The relatives need time to grieve, but you need to go off and start doing the paperwork. If it's a Jewish or Muslim one, I need to get somebody to do the death certificate immediately, so they can get the person buried by the following day. There's also other paperwork that has to be filled in, including who was on duty – you've got two hours and you need to get them over to the mortuary.

You haven't got time to think. It's a bit like when somebody goes into cardiac arrest on TV – the relatives are saying 'what's happening?' but the doctor is saying 'out of the way, I don't need your name, I just know that your heart has stopped and I need to get you breathing again'. You just get on with your job.

Discharge nurse 2

And occasionally, the unexpected can happen:

We had a Sikh gentleman who died and the family wanted him moved straightaway. They wanted to put him into the boot of the car. Our nurses found that very difficult – they really didn't want to help this family put this person in the boot of the car. The family were fine, but to us it wasn't fine. In the end, they put him in the back of the car. We did laugh about it afterwards. There are some differences in what we would find strange and what another culture does.

Head nurse

The next days

The next day or so, there are numerous practical things to be sorted by families. Hospice staff can be very helpful here:

Most people are very anxious to know what they have to do. I have little booklets with very good information, but it's not the same as someone sitting and talking it through with them. I do it quite slowly and method-ically and often write it all down. I give them the death certificate in an official envelope. I used to always seal the envelope, but now I don't – most people want to see what their loved one died of. Occasionally they're shocked, but that might be because of the medical terminology, so I talk to them quite directly.

I've got all the property and valuables here, very methodically lined up. We have our own bags. In the old days, we used a black bin liner, but I was not happy with that – it looked rather disrespectful. We are very careful about how people are treated at an extremely vulnerable time.

I will ask if they know how to get an undertaker. Many have no idea. We don't recommend one, but we know many local undertakers and have their cards. I would never just give one card, but four or five, so they can pick. I've learned who's quite good. There is one who is Irish, so if people are

from Ireland, I'd say they might find him helpful. Muslim undertakers
have their own procedures. Same with Jewish people.

My conversation can then lead into all kinds of things. Dying is quite
expensive, but money is quite delicate – you're not going to ask directly if
they have the money. A lot of people, after asking many other questions,
might ask how much it is going to cost. I always explain that the cost of a
very simple funeral is about £2,000. If they look aghast, I would then ask
if that is going to be a problem for them, because there is help available.
Social services used to pay for the whole funeral, but now they will only
contribute towards it. If the family refuse to pay or there is no next of kin
at all – and we've done many of those – then we hand everything over to
the local council and they do what used to be called a 'pauper's funeral'.
Now, thank God, it's a 'council funeral'.

You've got to be careful, because very often the people with clearly the
least money want a very grand funeral. Many people want a good show
and that is really important to them. They want a rosewood coffin with
golden handles and five cars – it can go up and up. We had a man not long
ago who said 'I don't care how much debt I get into, my father is having
the best funeral there ever was.' And he did. The son will be paying for it
for the next ten years.

Patient affairs officer

There is likely to be an effort to ascertain families' emotional needs as well:

The day after a death, we have a 'day after death meeting'. We invite the
families back and they collect the death certificate and we just do a mini
debriefing – how are they feeling? Was there anybody that needs to be
picked up with counselling at the moment? We like to leave people about
three months, so they can process what it is like to be without the person
that they have lost.

Counsellor 1

We have every background. Some are extremely reserved – they can just
walk in and nothing – no tears, nothing, very businesslike – 'my mother
died yesterday, have you got the death certificate ready?' I'm Irish and I'm
from a tradition where even as kids you were dragged around to every
local funeral. A wake and all that. So initially I was shocked that anybody
could be so very businesslike when they've just lost their wife, mother, or
whatever.

Patient affairs officer

This may be a time for a last viewing of the person who died:

Sometimes, families want to see the person again. When you're talking to
them, you do need to say 'when you touch them, they're going to be very

cold'. They've been in the fridge, but you don't say that, obviously! And people forget that and they touch them and they think gosh, they're really cold. So it's just getting used to that, more than anything else. A lot of people have some sort of fear, where they think the person is going to wake up again.

Counsellor 2

We get the person out of the storage facility and make sure that they're looking as best they can. That's the last time a relative is going to see their loved one and they need to be well presented. I usually ask the family how they want them to be dressed – sometimes the family will bring something in. I had a young girl who said she wanted to be buried in her Union Jack shorts. She was lovely. Sometimes we leave flowers on their pillow or a photograph of their wife. If they're Catholic, they like to have the rosary round their fingers. It's just paying attention to detail.

Senior staff nurse 1

Sometimes, families want to arrange for the person to be buried elsewhere:

We get a lot of people who relatives want to ship home, but they don't realise how expensive it is. It's most common with Africans. We had one woman who died and I think her church back home raised the funds to ship her home. None of the children knew that their mother was ill and that the father was coming back with her coffin. It is very hard, really.

Senior staff nurse 4

Nurses then complete a record of what happened:

We have a bereavement diary and, when a patient dies, we will write a bit of a story about the patient. It says when the patient came to us, what their stay was like and if there is any family. Sometimes we get family coming back and it's nice for them to look back, but it's more to help us to remember the patient. If family come a year later – and if there's nothing you can remember about the patient – it is embarrassing. Any member of staff can write in the book.

Senior staff nurse 3

Various arrangements exist to alert others around the hospice to a death, including people known to staff who died elsewhere:

When someone dies, we put up a poster in the centre with a generic statement which patients and staff came up with together, acknowledging that this person was a member of our community and, for the time that they were with us, we have enjoyed the experience of knowing them. And we acknowledge that their being with us was special. Then I put the name of the person and the date that they died and where they died. I put it up in the centre right by the main door. We also have a tall stool and we put a candle on the stool and a flower – that stays there for the first two days. People decided they didn't want a book of condolence.

If we know about a special friendship between patients, we will either contact that person when someone dies or I will meet with them as soon as they come in. And I'll sit with them in the office and talk about what's happened, so that they have a moment when they can manage that without being in the main room. Then they can make a decision about how they want the rest of the day to go.

Day centre manager

They've always had a system where a death notice is put up on the board in our volunteers' office. It will say when somebody died and if they died away from here. If they're day centre visitors and they died at home, I'll put something up about that as well. The volunteers know where to look.

Volunteer coordinator

And at the very end, there is the formal paperwork and other matters to be dealt with:

I have to notify the Healthcare Commission that we've had a death, so I get a copy of the form that they fill in to say that somebody's died. You look at that piece of paper as the end of somebody's life. I have to sign and send the form off.

If the death has been referred to the coroner, the coroner will only release the body once they're satisfied that there's nothing to investigate. This happens, for example, if someone hasn't been seen on a regular basis and dies very quickly. We had a patient whose family wanted her body to go back to her own country, but they were Jewish and wanted to have her buried within a certain time. It was a coroner's case and we're not allowed to take tubes out until the coroner says it's OK. So I had to ask the place where they register the death to be ready and we got a flight for that night. We had to do everything rapidly, so they could actually take her – we managed to do it.

Head of hospice 1

On rare occasions, there are problems which linger on after the death:

We had a woman some time ago who was drug dealing and, when she flew into the country, she went to prison. They found that she had advanced breast cancer and she came to us. The whole time she was here, our social work department were working hard to get her sons over here. She died with me on one of my night shifts. She's still in the mortuary now waiting for her sons to come over. No matter what she's done in her life, she must have been desperate and she's still not been reclaimed by her own family. It's horrendous.

Senior staff nurse 4

Attending funerals

There can be an issue for staff of whether they should attend the funeral of a patient who they cared for. Most say they do not, unless expressly invited:

> In the whole time since I have worked in palliative care, I have only gone to three funerals and that was because the relatives asked me and I had known them for about two years. But on the whole, it's unhealthy – you are here to do your job. You have to switch off when work is over.
>
> *Doctor 1*

> I don't go to funerals, because it is a family occasion. Occasionally the odd member of staff will go, if they know the person really well from outside or for many years. But personally, I wouldn't. I think we have got enough to cope with, with our own family when they die, than to try and cope with someone else's.
>
> *Nurse 1*

But there is the occasional exception:

> I have been to a few funerals if I am asked. I will only go to the service, I won't go back to the house or the social bit afterwards. That's their time. I have paid tribute to the person who has died and I've said my farewells. It's lovely listening to the eulogies. You hear such wonderful things about a person – you see a side that you never knew.
>
> *Senior staff nurse 2*

> I've been to a few funerals. Mostly where there's been no relatives. It's amazing how many people are living on their own without relatives. Like one Irish chap, he left no mark that he'd actually existed. He was living on his own – when he died, his only possessions were a suit, a television set and a radio. The priest said there was nobody to go the funeral and asked if I would go. It was very sad.
>
> *Volunteer 1*

It can be difficult to have a set policy:

> They discourage us from going to funerals, because they feel it is not good for us or the patients. But I don't think it is a good policy to forbid staff from going to funerals. Some feel that they say their goodbyes at a funeral. They may not have been on their shift when somebody they had become

close to dies, although for six weeks they had a lot to do with the patient and the family. All of a sudden there is nothing, they come in and there is an empty bed. So if somebody wants to go to a funeral, they should be allowed to.

Healthcare assistant 1

And sometimes, a hospice chaplain will be asked to officiate:

I am sometimes asked to do the funeral services for people here. I find it a very profound experience – being alongside a person who's in the last stages of their life and then being asked to take the service to say farewell. It feels the right place to be. When I am asked to conduct the service, that's the closure. And I'm offering this person to God in the name of Jesus – I have a sense of asking God to journey with this person beyond this life. It is quite special.

Chaplain 3

Bereavement work

The involvement of hospices with families does not always end with the death. They can be very attentive to the needs of relatives following a bereavement. Some people drop in when it is convenient:

A lot of families come back to see us. They've spent, say, two or three intense weeks here – and then all of a sudden their relative is gone and they don't have to come here anymore. I think they're very brave for coming in. It's hard because they can always pretend 'oh, I'm coming back, because they're still in that bed' – and they're not.

Senior staff nurse 4

And some families telephone for help:

We walk with people for as long as they need us by their side. It can be two years down the line and there will be a phone call from the family saying 'I'm going through a bit of a dip, can you help me?' They do come back and we help them the best way we can.

Chaplain 2

They have our contact numbers. Some people do pick up the phone for help, because one loss can sometimes trigger off a previous one which is unresolved. For example, there can be a mother who dies here, but you might find the father died only six months before and the children went from one crisis to the next. Somebody like that, we might pick up.

Counsellor 1

But hospices also have formal arrangements to invite families back for help, including counselling:

> Relatives are offered support long after their loved ones die. Families are invited to come back to what we call a 'bereavement tea', usually within six months. There are two a year – some will come to a couple and then not come back. They get together with the people they met here and the social workers. The volunteers will be around and I'm always there. They can also come to the social work team. So the palliative care continues – it's not just cut off when someone's body leaves here.
>
> *Volunteer coordinator*

> We run a group for bereaved spouses or partners. This takes place at the hospice and runs over a period of 12 weeks. Its purpose is to help people to cope with the change in their life. They meet other people who are experiencing similar feelings, so find it safe to explore events that have taken place. We also talk about the grieving process with them. People often feel they're going mad, because of some of the thoughts they have and some of the things they do – they glimpse someone in the street and think it is the person who has died or possibly lay a place at the table. It's about normalising this. It's OK, it's normal and you're not going mad.
>
> *Counsellor 2*

> We've had a couple of relatives who were determined to take their own life, but it doesn't happen very often. The longer you do the job, you get little alarm bells in your head and you say to yourself, 'this isn't quite right'. If I was worried about somebody, I'd put them onto the counsellors. You learn to read between the lines.
>
> *Senior staff nurse 1*

Bereavement work can also involve children:

> We run children's bereavement days. We have a programme of events to set them at their ease and to enable them to express their feelings in a way where it can be fun as well. So if a child wants to go into something in depth or is very distressed, that's all possible with a lot of support. But if a child wants to do it in a much more low key way, with the emphasis more on fun, that's possible as well.
>
> *Social worker*

Attention may be given to making a good place for relatives to visit:

> We've got a patient who's rung up and she said her family have collected some money and want to give us a bench. We get a lot of benches, some of them with inscriptions. That's something I'd like to get away from. The

families want to do something, but it's a bit in your face if you're dying and you're reading a plaque that said so-and-so died here. I'd like some kind of memorial wall, where people could come and sit, because we do get some people come back and they put flowers on.

Head of hospice 1

Subsequent contact with relatives

Because many families live locally to the hospice, it is not unknown for staff to meet them casually in the neighbourhood:

I bump into people in the street who say hello and ask how I am – and I'm thinking I don't know who they are. I now just reply 'I'm really well, thanks. Can you remind me, how do I know you?' And they laugh. Often they were families of patients from many years ago and they're with a new partner, a new family – you think that's great, they've moved on. And we've been part of that process, because if we hadn't offered the care and support after the death, some of them wouldn't get back on their feet at all.

Head of hospice 2

Relatives will see you in the high street and they expect you to remember them. What I normally say is 'your face is so familiar, but I can't remember your name for a minute' and as soon as they say something, often it triggers something. And they may go through the whole history of everything – and really you need to get to the bank before it closes. You're still a link to that dead person – it's trying to remember that. It might not be very convenient, but the bank will be open tomorrow.

Head nurse

But thoughts may linger on:

I stay in touch with very few families after someone has died. It's impossible because there are so many. Very often, I wonder how someone is doing. You've invested a huge amount of time and emotional energy and angst to achieve the thing and then the patient dies and that's it. Gone, let's get on with the next one. I've often wanted to go back to some families, when they've had a chance to reflect on this encounter and ask how did it affect them?

Consultant

PART II

DIFFICULTIES EXPERIENCED AND COPING WITH THEM

CHAPTER 6

Sources of stress: difficult patients and families

Most people would assume that working in a hospice is not easy. And, indeed, many nurses and others do not find it so. But some of the things which cause most difficulty might be surprising. This chapter explores one frequent source of problems: patients and relatives who are demanding, in denial or neglectful.

Difficult patients and relatives

Although nurses generally speak warmly about both patients and their families, there are many exceptions. Patients can be very demanding:

> We sometimes have challenging patients who feel that they're the only person who needs any help – that's very, very time consuming. We try to reason with them and if we can't, we just moan to each other in a quiet way, just to let off some steam. At the end of the day, it's not personal. Some will shout, some will swear and be quite abusive or they will just keep pressing the call bell – you may have just reset it and still be in the room and they'll re-press it. These things can really wear you down, because you're in a no-win situation.
>
> *Nina*

> You sometimes think they don't realise how many jobs we have to do. One night, a man who had dry skin was saying the nurses had not put cream over his body – I was on my hands and knees doing his legs at three o'clock in the morning. After I'd done that, there was something else he wanted. It's part of my job working here – you recognise that there will be a lot of demands on your time and your patience. You have to go along with that, because the next day they're not going to be here.
>
> *Helen*

Some people are simply difficult to like:

> We had one patient who was particularly trying – it wasn't her illness, but her personality. And I thought 'I really don't like you' and then I felt guilty thinking it. I spoke to one of the senior nurses later about this and she said

'it is OK not to like somebody'. And after that, I thought well, I am a human being and if there is a difficult situation, I have to step back and ask not to go into that room for a bit. It doesn't happen very often.

Fiona

Perhaps more often, relatives are very demanding on behalf of a patient:

Some relatives think we're stupid. We had a patient whose son used to phone up at 4.00 in the morning asking if I had changed her oxygen cylinder. You have people who feel that their mother is the most important person in the world. Obviously, they are to them, but they need to see that we've got someone else who's a very special person to someone else. And standing there staring at me doesn't mean I'm going to get that painkiller any quicker.

Rebecca

One relative complained that a patient hadn't had a wash for a couple of days. But when I looked through the notes, it was because the patient had refused one. We try to respect the patient's wishes. If they're not going to come to any harm by not having a wash, that might be their last chance to say no and it's not for us to take it away. Some families find that difficult.

Nina

Some relatives are not happy about the medication. They feel we are sedating the patient or that the medication is making them worse. I've been told to take syringe drivers down from people who are dying, because the family believes that it is not medicine. That is problematic, because you are putting the patient at risk of discomfort.

Michelle

Some demands seem particularly unreasonable:

We had one patient where I set up carers to go into their home to give personal care, but the family wanted their washing doing, their cooking, their cleaning – they even expected the carers to wash the doorstep. And when they didn't get this, they were ringing me back saying 'it is all falling apart'. The son was abusive to me. I found that very stressful.

Discharge nurse 1

Demands on hospice staff can begin even before a patient gets to the hospice:

I recently received a referral for a gentleman who's terminally ill. I checked the location and it came up for a health authority we do not have a contract with, which means we will not be paid for it. I just put 'declined, not in our area', pointed out other hospices they could apply to and thought that was the end of it. I then got a telephone call from the patient's daughter saying 'I'm appealing to your compassion. If you say no, that means my father will die alone', because she lives and works near here. It was just more convenient for her. I tried to explain that my compassion is not a deciding factor on admission to here. I felt annoyed, because my job should involve dealing only with professional referrers.

Discharge nurse 2

Anger and aggression

In addition to being generally difficult, some patients can become very aggressive:

There have been people here that were very threatening. Some have led very shambolic lives – and that's not going to change just because they're in here. So we've certainly had people here being extremely rude, telling me to F-off. I'd just say they don't need to speak to me like that.

Louise

We never know enough about patients who come here. The doctors used to go to the home to see the patient before they came in, but sometimes they just come straight into here. Sometimes, we will find that they are life threatening to themselves or to us. We found out that one patient had burnt his house down. We thought 'whoops, that's nice to know'. And we have the occasional patient in handcuffs, their prison officer is with them. It feels a bit edgy – you are scared to go in the room especially on night duty, because you don't know what's going to happen. It is not so bad after you get to know them.

Dan

This anger can also be displayed by people in the day centre:

Sometimes people walk in the room like they have a black cloud over their heads. I tend to alert the staff, encouraging them to pay attention to it, but not do anything, unless it looks like they're going to have a go at someone. We try to ask as gently as possible what they are feeling so angry about. Sometimes touching someone when they're in distress shifts the dynamic.

If I hear a yell and, even if it seems like a yell in fun, I'll walk into the main room and see what's going on. It makes people feel safer knowing that I or another staff member will come and manage any situation. If people see conflict and don't see it resolved, they're left feeling incredibly anxious, so we always try to show situations being resolved.

The weather, especially in the winter, is important. People are coming in the dark, going home in the dark, it's a bad time of year – lots of people have Seasonal Affective Disorder. If people are getting grumpy, I urge staff not to respond to it, but just to recognise what's happening and maybe even start a conversation saying 'no wonder you're feeling bad, it's the winter, it's horrible'. Now that might not be the reason, but it's a safe way of beginning a conversation about how they are feeling.

Day centre manager

Relatives can also become aggressive or abusive:

Every nurse here will tell you that she's finished her shift in tears at some point. You think you've really done your best and then something's happened and everything falls to pieces. We had a gentleman in – the wife was a professional woman of some kind, used to saying her bit. She wasn't grasping that he was dying and I was trying to be honest and she completely blasted me down at the top of her voice. I can't remember exactly what she said, but just that I obviously had no idea what I was talking about – she was a very articulate woman, so she was able to just blast me with vocabulary. Luckily the manager overheard everything and told her that she couldn't speak to staff like that and she was asked to leave.

Rebecca

I have had very few people who have raised their voice to me. One was the son of a lady who was terminally ill. When she realised that her time was coming very close, she said she wanted to go home. We knew that she would be lucky to see the day out, double checked that this was really what she wanted and proceeded to set it up for her. We couldn't get hold of her son, but as she was being taken by the ambulance men out of the building, he came in the door.

Before anyone could explain to him, he just went for somebody in a uniform and it was me. I was a bit shaken up. He was just beside himself with grief, his mum was dying, he didn't know that she had wanted to go home. He was saying 'how stupid can you be sending my mother home, she is dying!' I tried to guide him into a room, so that his mum wouldn't hear him. A couple of family members were trying to calm him down. I said 'it is OK, I know that it is not directed at me, it is because of what's going on'. People's emotions are very, very high. Who knows what I might be like, if it happened to me?

Fiona

Very occasionally, anger can escalate to physical aggression:

Patients can strike out. One night, a patient was drinking on his medica-tion, which makes you really highly strung. All of a sudden, every bell went off in one go. We were rushing to the different bells to find this patient frightening the others. I got him out of one patient's room and thought that was the end of it. And then out of the corner of my eye, I saw him come back into the room and he took my throat and pushed me against the wall – I was being strangled. I managed to push him away and we got the charge nurse to get him back into his room.

When the morning staff came on, the patient said he couldn't remember a thing. When we came in that night, there was an enormous box of chocolates, as a way of saying sorry. But I said 'I am not accepting the apology, he shouldn't be on this ward, he frightened the staff'. It is very difficult when you have been frightened badly.

Dan

One of the first things I ever got called to in the hospice was a patient who assaulted the doctor – really lashed out at him. The doctor was doing his rounds early in the morning and the patient just turned on him. He was quite bruised afterwards – it was his private parts that got hit, so it was pretty horrific. I got bleeped and went running down. The doctor was sitting in a chair, really shaken and startled, but he was OK. The patient was all over the place, throwing stuff around and trying to wreck his room. We calmed him down and called the police, who took him away. I felt everybody else was at risk and we needed to make the hospice safe for the majority of patients. He wasn't at risk. I think he had been out drinking the night before – we were more lax then about letting respite patients go out. We're a bit stricter now.

Head of hospice 1

There are many differing reasons for such anger. Many relatives are simply angry at the situation they are in, coupled with a lot of exhaustion:

The people who give the most trouble are often those who have not come to the terms with what's wrong with their loved one. We've had a few who have been unbelievably difficult. They complain, they interfere, they throw tantrums about their mother or father – usually it's a parent – and the care they're getting. They are obviously just trying every means possible.

Jill

It's a very stressful time. Relatives may have been looking after somebody for a long time without any support. There will come a point where the carer just can't take any more – they haven't slept well for ages, they haven't eaten well, they haven't socialised. They haven't really been part of the human race for quite a long time. Then when the patient comes here, it may be very difficult to hand over the care to somebody whom they don't know, or even trust. They may find it frustrating if the patient's needs aren't met as quickly as they would like.

Eileen

There may be anger at earlier treatment:

> Our contacts with people are short and very intense. Often, we pick up not only the patients, but their families when they're terribly angry and resentful. You get the butt of their anger against the rest of the medical profession – they always refer to things that have gone wrong, rather than the things that have gone right. You get mad about it and then you talk to your colleagues, just like anything else.
>
> *Consultant*

Some people may feel very let down by others:

> People have expectations of other people. There might be two sisters with a mother dying and one copes well with the caring role and the other finds she can't do that, but she can do the paperwork. Then, the first sister complains that the other never comes to the hospice – 'she doesn't do this, she doesn't do that'. And we have to say we're all different – what you can cope with is different. Some people are fearful of people dying. So where families have got on quite well, all of a sudden they disintegrate because their expectations of each other are unrealistic. It's all very well saying 'she should be here for our mother', but some people just cannot do that.
>
> I try to get families together to talk about expectations. They tend to come to a point where they will work together as best they can. They may never talk to each other afterwards – that's entirely up to them. But what we want to do is try to make it OK for the patient. They have the time to sit there and think about things. Mostly it works. People tend to realise that they need to put their own stuff on hold – that they need to put the patient first.
>
> *Counsellor 2*

And some will have been angry with each other for a long time:

> Some families have, for want of a better word, 'baggage' that they haven't dealt with. Maybe they haven't had a good relationship and it's now come to the boil. They take it out in different ways, but some are quite difficult. You can't take it personally – you've got to try to find a way through. If you do it well, it's great. When you don't, you do reflect on it, if there was anything to learn for the next occasion. You've got to appreciate that you're not going to get it 100% right. You can't solve 50 years of baggage in a week!
>
> *Catherine*

We nurse the family, rather than just one person. That can often be very challenging, especially if you get a dysfunctional family where one person isn't talking to another. You have to have the same conversation four or five times and sometimes they don't agree. The family dynamics can be tiring. We can't put too much energy into resolving problems that have been there for 30 years. Sometimes, these are long-standing family feuds and you need to learn to accept, for your own peace of mind, that you can't solve everything.

Jessica

There are both informal and formal ways of dealing with people who became too aggressive:

If something has gone wrong, you're the butt because you happen to be there at the time – it really isn't personal and they will feel as bad about it as you do. Sometimes you need to be very direct and say 'I know you're very angry – why don't we sit down and have a look at what the problem is'. Quite often, as soon as they sit down, there will be tears and they will just let it go. And then maybe we will talk and talk, because really it's just pent up anger and frustration.

Eileen

We developed a behavioural contract for patients. If they have a problem with their behaviour, we would write it down and we'd contract with them not to do that – and if they did, we'd give them so many chances and then that would be it. We have had some that we've refused admission, because they didn't stick to the contract. This has helped the staff.

Head of hospice 1

Patients and families in denial

Staff clearly have difficulties when anger or aggression is directed at them. But they can also find it difficult to watch patients or relatives who will not acknowledge – and therefore deal with – the proximity of death:

There are some relatives who can't accept what is happening. We have the same conversations over and over. They will ask a question to one nurse and then another. They may say their mum hasn't had anything to eat and why is she not eating? We try to explain that the personal need for food just goes, but they insist she should be eating and then go and find every nurse on the shift and ask the same question. Some don't accept it until their relative has actually died – 'they were fine and they come in here and two weeks later she's dead'.

We had a patient recently and she knew she was dying, she just didn't want to acknowledge it. She'd say 'when I'm out of here, I need to get some things for my grandchild' – and this woman had the hugest breast tumour you've ever seen, completely swollen up, she couldn't move. We told her that she was very poorly and if she wanted to go down the high street to pick up some things for her grandchild, she shouldn't wait – we would get her in a wheelchair and do it the next day. She did get tearful and looked at me and said 'I need you to keep my hope alive'. It's difficult. If I don't know what to say, I just don't say anything or I say that I don't know what to say to you, I'm sorry.

Rebecca

Some people don't recognise that they're ill. I asked one patient at home with a massive tumour what she thought it was, 'oh it's nothing, don't worry about it'. It was a breast tumour that was smelling, it was obvious and she was refusing anyone to go in. She said I didn't need to visit her, but she lived alone. In the end, I referred her back to her GP. There wasn't much more that I could do. I can't force patients to accept our care.

Community nurse

People may say they are getting better or discuss what they will do next year, but what they're actually doing is saying 'I wish'. There are people who are seriously in denial as well – if they don't want to talk, we're not going to push it. We will look at what's troubling them now. And we will try to say, in some way, perhaps there are some things they need to be looking at.

Eileen

Denial can also affect patients' expectations of further treatment:

When families want to continue treatment, you just have to work your way through it. Sometimes even with a full explanation, families will still deny. Legally, we don't have to do anything that we feel is damaging to a patient, but it's like all things, you want to negotiate and reach an understanding. But you've got to be prepared to put time in to do it, because it can some-times take a long time to win people round. Time is the resource that is in all too short supply and yet it is the resource that will ultimately help solve those problems.

Consultant

I had a lady at home who was obviously dying, but the family wouldn't stop any treatment, so they were giving her fluids through a drip which was going straight into her chest. She was bringing up secretions and the family asked if we could give her something to dry them up. I said we could, but it would be defeating the object of giving her fluids. I explained that she was terminal and there weren't many benefits to the fluids, as they were actually causing her distress, but they wouldn't hear of it. Until she took her last breath, they were giving her these injections and I just thought that was a shame, because she could have died much more peacefully.

Community nurse

In some cases, each person is trying to protect the other:

> You often get the scenario where the patient will appear to not know what's going on, so the family won't talk about it, but if you pull them all apart, they are all protecting each other. You get 'I don't think mum knows that she is dying', but then you talk to mum and she knows full well exactly what's happening, but she doesn't want to tell the children, because she doesn't want to upset them. That's where we can unravel it a bit. I will ask the mother how it would be for her if she told her daughter, there may be things left unsaid. Quite often, it doesn't take very much, it is just somebody making that first move. We all try the British stiff upper lip, 'I am not really in a hospice, I am not really that ill'. None of us want to accept we are going to die.
>
> *Claire*

Denial is felt to be particularly hard on children, whether young children or somewhat older:

> I have known children in their early teens who had not been prepared for a parent's death. The family wouldn't let us do any counselling work with any of them. They kept control of the situation by not letting anybody in, 'we are all right, we are fine'. But nobody was saying that she was going to die – we could see that, but they were absolutely adamant they didn't want any help. And they weren't fine at all – those children were absolutely distraught. They weren't prepared for it in any way, shape or form.
>
> *Claire*

> The most difficult cases are the ones with children. Parents will keep putting off telling them the truth about what is happening, because they don't want them to worry. But children worry all the way through. Children notice the changes, whatever they are, and actually deal with it so much better, because they've not got all the baggage adults have. We can do some fantastic work with youngsters if we're allowed to talk to the family. We can explain about memory boxes, letters, mementoes. Whereas if they're not told, they can become very distressed after the death and feel they have missed out on things they wanted to say. It's about feeling abandoned, of being left with no preparation. Unfortunately, it does happen a lot.
>
> *Counsellor 2*

Such problems can be made more complicated where staff are unclear what patients are being told:

> I've got a Bengali lady whose husband sees her dying, but won't tell her because he thinks it will upset her. She doesn't speak very much English.

She's got ovarian cancer, she's going to know and I said that to him, but he won't have it – they've got very young children and he won't tell them either. When I visit, he tends to put them in the other room. I don't know what he's telling them, but there's nothing I can do. I'm trying to get an interpreter in, but he still won't have her told that she's dying. I think she has a right to know, because she may want to talk to her children and her children might want to talk to her about dying – and she's not given the opportunity to do that. It is sad when that happens.

Community nurse

Denial has been known to happen even after a death:

A lady came in here and her husband died – they were both in their thirties – and from the day of diagnosis, she just would not have it. She had only been married for about five years. We had to literally, bodily, take her out of the room. She kept saying 'he is going to wake up, he is going to wake up' and we were trying to be gentle, saying 'no, you have been in here a couple of hours, please come away'. In the end, someone had to say to her 'he is dead, he is gone, you cannot bring him back' – they had to be quite firm with her, because otherwise she would have just laid there with him all night. That's distressing, when somebody is absolutely heartbroken.

Fiona

Not everyone feels that denial should be seen as a problem:

We went through a stage of thinking everybody has to come to terms, but I don't think we have got the right to do that. If people can't handle the news, that's fine, then we work with them. Often, the patient knows full well what they are doing. I don't think anybody really wakes up on a Wednesday morning and dies at 11 o'clock and hasn't had any inkling. I think they know, but they don't say it.

Carole

I try to gauge what they really know and if they really don't want you to speak about it, why should we force it on them? It might be their way of saying 'that's enough, thanks. I've had everything else done to me'. You have to let people have as much control of their life as they can. They've lost their role in the family, they may feel they're losing dignity, because they can't wipe their own bottom anymore. You just have to pick up on the cues in case they change their mind. Listening is important. Not just listening, but hearing and understanding and not putting your own interpretation on something.

Nina

Family neglect

In addition to the angry families and the protective families, there are also those who do not give sufficient attention to the person who is dying. This can also be distressing:

> I remember one family, the daughter couldn't wait for her mother to die, to get her out of her life, because she was too much of a nuisance. The grandson always said 'how's my gran?' and he was interested, but the daughter couldn't wait for her to go. You just have to deal with it, you just have to carry on talking to them.
>
> *Dan*

> One woman had been living with her son and his wife. It was terribly distressing because we began to feel that his motives in relation to her were to do with money – he just did not visit her here. There was one occasion when the doctor phoned him to come in quickly, because she was very, very ill, and he said he was in the middle of a meeting and would have to phone back. She so wanted her son to come and see her and she talked and talked about him. He came for half an hour one day and then not after that.
>
> The last time I talked to her, we sat and I held her hand and we talked about things and she never mentioned her son once – not once. I realised that she had come to some resolution and she knew he wasn't coming. She said 'you've all helped me so much here, it's been lovely being here' and I just thought we have to be thankful that she felt that she had that. He came after she'd died and sat with her for two hours, crying and saying how lovely she was.
>
> *Anna*

Very occasionally, families are too eager for a death to occur:

> We had one family, who was Jewish. The son arranged for the undertakers to pick his mother up on the Sunday, because if she had died on a Friday, she would have had to stay in the room. He had arranged her funeral before she even died. The funeral was supposed to be on the Sunday and she was still here on the following Wednesday. We were going 'oh, I don't believe this is happening'. The son that arranged that died six months later himself.
>
> *Dan*

CHAPTER 7

Other sources of stress and their impact

The previous chapter outlined some of the difficulties faced by hospice staff arising from different demands from patients and their relatives. This chapter explores some difficulties of other kinds, including an emotional involvement with patients and various pressures of work, and their effect on staff and their families.

Emotional involvement

For a variety of reasons, hospice nurses and others can become very emotionally attached to some patients. This seems to be common:

> There are some people you get closely involved with, because you see them quite frequently. When you work through a difficult situation, you get to know them quite well, even in a very short space of time. You learn a lot about them and you can get quite emotionally attached to them, but you can't allow that to happen all the time – otherwise you'd never do anything.
>
> *William*

> I do get close to some patients. It's difficult not to. Sometimes it makes me go more than the extra mile. You stay longer – you just want to be around for them. And when you're on your way out, relatives may come in and they want to talk to you and you think you'd better talk to them.
>
> *Grace*

> There is an attachment that occurs, a level of intimacy that you get around death. People will be really open with you. People think that they really like you, but it is just because you have opened yourself up to each other and there is a bond there.
>
> *Michelle*

It may be the relatives whose pain is most difficult to take:

> It isn't the patients that get to me, it's the relatives. When patients have died, their suffering has finished. The relatives are carrying on – you do

empathise with certain people and it may be the ones you least expect. It can affect you, even ten years down the line.

Nina

There are some who you become closer to – you have something that they open up to. There was a gentleman who would visit his wife every day, and you knew he was going home to this empty house. He would just come and sit and sit in the reception. I did offer him a lift home once. I haven't had many like that.

Dorothy

Where staff are dealing with a patient dying at home, there are particular issues:

A death means that the next time I go into the house, I will just see the relative or the partner. It feels strange, because obviously the presence of the patient is now not there, they're not sitting there – you walk in and it's a bit eerie, because your focus is different, you are there to support.

Community nurse

Very young patients affect some people particularly strongly:

If someone's old, it's a little more acceptable, because they've had their life. It's different if you have someone who's 26 and who has a really full life ahead of them. If they just got married or they've just had a child, I find that quite difficult to deal with. The whole team does as well, it affects the whole atmosphere.

Charlotte

Thank God, we don't get too many very young people here. In general, the younger they are, the harder it is to be philosophical about it. If someone dies and they're 85 and their family are here and they die very peacefully, you can say he had a good life, he's seen his children, he's seen his grandchildren, he didn't suffer – not bad.

Louise

But some argue that elderly patients are equally affecting, particularly where they have been married for a long time:

Age makes no difference at all. There can be somebody who's really elderly who's just so lovely. Sometimes that's harder, because the families have had these people for so long, they think they are going to have them for ever. There is no good scenario, really. Everybody's grief is completely individual, whether the patient is 35 or 95 – they are a human being who's dying.

Claire

I find it very upsetting when elderly people pass away, especially when they have a partner, because they may have been married for 60 years. The person who is left is so alone. It must be like losing their right arm. Sometimes, there will be a poor little old lady, maybe in her late eighties and her husband is dying and you think 'God, what's going to happen to you?'

Fiona

There may be concern that too strong an emotional attachment can affect the ability to give good care:

You can get too close. If your own sadness prevents you from being there to support the family, then you probably won't be the right person to give professional support. Sometimes you may have something in common, but you should be on the level that you can support the family. If you're not, then it's important that you recognise it.

Julia

There's only one patient I couldn't care for – he reminded me of my uncle both in the way he looked and in some of his mannerisms. One of my colleagues looked after him. My uncle is well, but it worried me. I just didn't think I could be making judgements professionally. It was a bit too close to home.

Vicky

Questions arise about the extent to which nurses should show their emotion when patients to whom they feel close become very ill or die:

When I trained, there was this big thing in nursing about you weren't supposed to get upset if a patient died. But I might have nursed this person for a month and that would be a month of getting to know the family – they deserve to see that I cared enough to get a bit upset. I won't collapse and cry in front of them, but I will let them know that I am a bit upset. The time I don't care about at least one person in that way is possibly the time I shouldn't be here.

You have to maintain a certain amount of empathy and a certain amount of compassion, but be able to control it. I have a cry, have a quick fag and then you move on. It's when you're not moving on when the trouble starts – when you are not able to step back. This isn't your family and you need to respect the boundary.

Jessica

Something will hit you out of the blue. You are fine and all of a sudden, you think 'oh my God, I am going to cry, I had better go out'. It might be the patient looking at you and you can't do anything else for them. Or you might get somebody stroking a relative's hand or whispering something in their ear – you would have to be as hard as nails not to feel choked. And you will say to them 'maybe it is time to say goodbye now' and they will do that.

I don't think it is wrong for the relatives to see you sad, because if you stood there with a smile on your face saying it is OK – it would not be normal. I've put my arms around relatives and my eyes have filled up, but I have never lost control. If I thought I was going to, I would go out of the room – there is always a bathroom. I have put my head in my hand and sobbed.

Fiona

Some find themselves letting out pent-up emotion outside the hospice:

Before I started here, I had no experience of motor neurone disease, where the mind is so alert and the body just fails you completely. One day, I asked a patient 'is there anything I can do for you before I leave the room?' and he said 'could you scratch my nose?' And that day, I drove home and I sobbed all the way home. I just thought how can there be a God, when somebody has to suffer? It will hit you just when you don't expect it.

Claire

Sometimes it's the little tiny things that make me cry. One time, we'd had a really busy day and a patient died quite late in the shift. I felt that there had been one thing after another. I went home and poured myself a glass of milk and burst into tears – I was crying for a good while. But afterwards, I felt much better. That happens at times.

Julia

A very elderly lady who I had known as a friend came in here very short term and died. I'd known her a long time, her death was expected, she was a very elderly lady, almost 90, but when I went home, I just sat down and tears flowed. I realised that her passing was cathartic – perhaps it released all the unshed tears about everybody else. It became an honouring of everybody's life – it wasn't really her particularly who I was crying for. It just allowed everything to flow.

Alice

The death of a colleague can affect hospice staff as a group:

Julian, our Head Nurse died recently. We all knew him very well. He died of cancer and must have known his symptoms. We were told he was very ill – we didn't know if he was going to come back to work or not – and then, out of the blue, we were told that he had died. That knocked the sails out of all of the staff. The funeral service was just a terrible day, because literally every staff member was in tears. Most of us went to the funeral.

We still keep thinking 'oh, is he coming through the door?' His heart's still with us.

Dan

That's the only time in all the years I've been here that I literally folded up. He was very funny, but also very shy. He could drive you mad like everybody else, but he was extremely easy to be around. He just made it a fun place to work. It was devastating to lose him. He left here early one day and said he an appointment at the hospital. I knew he hated hospitals and doctors, like all of us who work here. And off he went, smiled, bye. Later, I rang his mobile and he said 'you're not going to believe it, they have me in bed – they're doing tests'. He wouldn't let anybody see him, which was quite hard. I wrote to him every day, sent cards, begged him to let me come, because then we knew it was bad.

The hospice was fantastic. They did everything they could possibly do. They knew it had a devastating effect on everybody, particularly the people who knew him a long time. There's still a big fallout from it. About two days ago, a patient walked in and I said 'isn't it amazing, that man was meant to die eight years ago and Julian was so helpful to him – and there he is, doing very well, and Julian's dead'.

Louise

Julian died of cancer – he shouldn't get cancer, we're the carers. So there was a shock – it was massive. He walked out one August day and said 'I'll see you Monday' and he sent a text over the weekend to say he was having a couple of investigations – and that's the last we ever saw of him. We felt deserted, as though he walked out and left. He was a real character and very lovable. His death was very quick. We sent presents, we sent flowers, but there was no contact – and that's what we couldn't cope with.

We had a memorial service, designed by some of the patients and staff. Some got up and told stories and it was fantastic. We involved the family in the planning. On the anniversary, we had an afternoon tea and just spent a few minutes remembering him. The family turned up and presented us with a photograph of him and showed us old pictures of him. I suppose it was a bit like closure, it had all come to an end.

Catherine

Particular frustrations

Some of the difficulties of hospice work arise from the very nature of the work undertaken. The most obvious is dealing with very ill people and, sometimes, a lot of deaths:

If you are with a patient for a long time and they have a lot of needs, it can stress you out. Sometimes you can't sort something out – you do your best, but you can't always do everything. And they get frustrated, so by the time you come out of that room, you are so stressed.

Dan

Sometimes the going does get tough, when you've had a particularly hard week, for instance a lot of deaths or really complicated patients who have demanded a lot of time and energy. Some people just need a lot of input. If you have a few of those in one week, that can be quite taxing.

Charlotte

It does take your energy if you have a few people dying closely together. We need to get on with the work – and sometimes it seems that there's no time to stop in between. It does have an effect on the staff.

Julia

But there are also other sources of frustration. This may be dealing with other agencies:

I get frustrated with social services. I can't do big adaptations because of the time it takes. If someone's relatively well, I might consider referring them, but there's a waiting list of about 18 months for a stair lift so for a lot of my patients, that is not appropriate. If someone really wanted one and they had the means, I would give them information on purchasing one privately. If not, you have to consider downstairs living, which isn't always appropriate.

I can't make special orders for things, because that could take a month and by the time it comes, the person may well have deteriorated and not be able to use it. It's really frustrating. I needed a lap tray to help a lady who was bed-bound to sit up and read and write. They didn't have that in their standard stock, so I ordered one – it ended up taking six weeks and by that time, she'd died.

Occupational therapist

You could sit down and work out the most perfect arrangements for home care and you think you've covered everything – transport home, oxygen, somebody there for the patient, first person going in. But as soon as someone leaves, it's out of your hands. I deal with social services and they contract the work out to a care agency, so it gets moved further out of your control. Sometimes a few months later the chap's back in again, because it's not working – the carers are not turning up or they're not really doing anything.

Discharge nurse 2

Or coping with complaints of one kind or another:

We get the occasional complaint. One lady, whose mother died at 93 three years ago, hasn't accepted it. She reported us to the General Medical

Council, saying that the doctor killed the patient, but they wouldn't enter-tain it. She reported the staff to the Nursing and Midwifery Council – they looked at it and said there was nothing. She reported us to the police and they came and said there was nothing. The Healthcare Commission have come on a number of occasions and gone thoroughly through the records, met me, interviewed staff and she's still not going to accept it. We've tried to get her to come in and talk to us. I feel sorry for her. She's at war with the world and it's a shame that she hasn't found peace. It is sad her mum died, but she died a very peaceful death. It's been a learning experience being investigated and having to write reports. At the end of the day, you've got to get past it.

Head of hospice 1

Sometimes, staff have said something which was not appropriate or done something that wasn't quite sensitive. We go and talk with the upset rela-tives or friend. Very occasionally we have allegations, people who say 'so and so was rough when they handled me' – and that obviously needs to be investigated. The staff member concerned will be asked to describe what they did that day, what they think the person meant. Sometimes it needs to go a little higher, just to talk things over, 'did you understand that this is what the person was saying?' It's just basically talking. People don't always understand how someone else can perceive something.

Eileen

I had a chap who had had a carer in his home and he felt that one or two things had gone missing from his flat – quite serious accusations. I arranged a meeting with the patient, social services, the agency that the social services had contracted out to and the girl who was giving the care. It turned out that it was the boyfriend who used to visit when she was at work. My responsi-bility was then to make sure that when my patient went home, he had a new carer who was monitored very closely on a weekly basis.

Discharge nurse 2

Senior staff can find it difficult to help more junior staff with their problems:

Quite often, nurses will come to me with personal things – they need to change their off duty time and they may not want to tell everybody why. Or they will have a worry with another member of staff, whether personal or professional. They may feel that someone isn't performing well and it's not been picked up. I look at whether it is a perceived underperformance or an actual underperformance – it can be difficult, but I see a lot. If I feel there is a problem, I will speak to the nurse involved and we would look at strategies to change that behaviour.

It's hard coping with nurses' private problems. You know them person-ally, you empathise with them personally as a friend and colleague. But as

> a manager, you have to think about how something will affect the rest of the staff or, indeed, the care of patients, because if staff leave it is a problem. The higher you go, the wider the effects are going to be.
>
> *Head nurse*

In addition, the occasional person may feel that other staff do not understand what they contribute:

> Counselling isn't always understood. There are some times when I can feel the nurses wonder what counsellors actually do. I try to explain, but it is an invisible service. I don't put sticking plasters all over a person and say 'that one's mended emotionally'. I find that difficult. People are distressed because the person they love is dying – I can't make them stop crying just because I am a counsellor.
>
> *Counsellor*

> I feel sometimes that some of the staff don't always understand the pressures of my job. They'll say 'she's sitting at the computer again, what's she doing all day?' without realising everything else that goes on. One actually said she wondered what I did, but then when I was away, she found out exactly what I had to do. You don't see what another person's job entails until you have to do it.
>
> *Head nurse*

General pressures of work

In addition to the many difficulties shown, there can be general pressures of work. These can arise in any profession, but tend to have a particular poignancy in this context. People can feel there is not enough time to do the job well:

> There have been days when we have been particularly busy. There was one day where I took myself round the back of the hospice and sat on the grass and cried my eyes out, I was so frustrated. We didn't have enough staff, there was staff sickness, it was the summer. This particular day, there was one patient where we could not get on top of her pain. I felt she deserved better. I kept saying 'please, somebody give this lady pain relief'. It wasn't their fault, there were so many people who needed things and there weren't enough nurses to go round, but the frustration was immense. Later, I said 'we failed that lady – she was in pain for over an hour, because nobody could get to her'. That's very, very rare.
>
> *Fiona*

> It's almost a conveyor belt you're on – people come, they die and there's someone to take their place. And if I think about that, I get distressed, because I feel this intense relationship, they die, they're gone, you never

see the family again – and that's really sad. They're gone and someone else takes their place. There's very little time to sit back and reflect.

William

The long hours can be very tiring:

> I work 12 hour shifts, so I come in at 7.30 in the morning and work till 8.30 and the night shift will run from 8.00 pm until 8.00 am. Most of us don't get out in time on a fairly regular basis, particularly when we're very busy. Sometimes, it can be an hour that we stay after the shift has ended.
>
> *Eileen*

> I'm contracted to do 30 hours, but I often do a 12- or 14-hour day when we've got groups and supervision. On Monday, I always say to my husband 'I'm only doing a half day today' and he says 'your half day is everybody's working day'. I would come in on a Sunday for maybe three or four hours.
>
> I'm on call 24/7. I don't get called much, but it varies. I sometimes get home and get a call and have to go back out again. It's all according to which nursing staff are on duty and how experienced they are. They would call me if someone needs a counsellor. I'd check if there's another way we can work it, but it could be that somebody's dying and part of the family may have just arrived and they're in pieces and feel they need to see a counsellor.
>
> *Counsellor 2*

And it can be difficult to stop thinking about particular patients or work in general:

> I get quite tired and then I can't switch off. When I work until 9.00 at night, I will get home at 10.00, but I probably won't fall asleep till midnight. Your mind just races around everything you've done that day. You remember something someone said to you. It's very difficult to calm down, but you desperately want to, because you've got to be up at 6.00 the next morning.
>
> *Rebecca*

> This week, we had a lady die here and lots of people turned up to view her body. Apart from being physically exhausting, it was quite emotional. You can't speak to each person individually, which is what I would have liked to have done. And then I had some complex things on the ward to deal with as well, so I just felt as if I had done a week's work in one day. It can be a lot to process. I have gone home two nights and not wanted to do very much. I just needed to be quiet because physically, I was tired and mentally, I was exhausted.
>
> *Claire*

If you have a long day, then a day off, and another long day, you can't really do much in between, so you are more or less trying to relax as much as you can. It is very difficult to blank things out, especially if something has upset you. It can be very difficult to unwind from a patient passing away. Sometimes when you are having a bath, you will let it go out, your emotions fall down and you cry.

Dan

Some find it hard to work nights:

We do what is called a week of nights, which is seven days from 8.30 at night till 8.00 in the morning – we do seven nights on and seven days off. It is hard to pull your body clock round, sleeping during the day. Then when you have finished doing a week of nights, trying to pull your body clock back round again can take a week or more. A few people prefer to do regular nights, because they have got used to doing night after night.

Dan

I don't do very well at night – I prefer days. I don't mind working an odd night, but when I've got a couple strung together, I don't sleep very well during the day. I then get quite scared coming to work because I hope I don't get irritable with one of the patients.

Laura

And there is always the fear that stress and over-tiredness will lead to a mistake:

There was a point where I was at burnout. It came about because of a particular lady. She was unconscious and her daughters wanted her to be given fluids and it really wasn't going to be to her benefit, but we facilitated absolutely everything that they wanted. The lady died and they then accused us of euthanasia. We offered them a post mortem and they said no – the accusations just went on and on. And for the first time in my life, I felt like saying to her 'why the hell don't you listen to what we're saying?' I was so close to saying it, it scared me. I really felt we'd given our all and it wasn't enough – I didn't want to do this anymore. I went on holiday for two weeks and when I came back, I was better. I had recharged my batteries and could come back and be quite objective.

Nina

I remember coming in on a Monday morning and there were six deaths over the weekend. That is a lot to deal with. It's also the easiest time in the world to make a big mistake. Six deaths, six lots of property, you could give somebody the wrong things. It's never happened, but I had one near miss. The phones were ringing, people were coming in and rushing me and I nearly did it! And I learned. I thought I will never be rushed, ever. You have to get that one completed and then move on to the next one – you've got to be meticulous.

Patient affairs officer

At a minimum, it can be difficult not to show patients the degree to which staff are rushing:

There's never enough time. You're always chasing your tail. You're sort of running and then you go and talk to them and you slow right down. Then you get up slowly and you run round to the next one, then you slow right down. You don't want them to think that you're busy and you can't spend time with them. It would be awful to think that they didn't want to bother us, because we're busy.

Laura

The impact on staff and their families

As might be expected, people's health can be affected by the pressures of their work:

There can be days of patients and relatives and members of staff needing your attention constantly from 9 to 5 on the phone and doing visits. I once had five deaths in two weeks. I was exhausted. I just didn't know where I was going. I don't have that many days off sick, but I do feel a tightness in my chest. I notice that when I'm getting stressed, my cheeks hurt and my eyes get a bit lazy, so that for me is an indicator that I need to look at what's going on around me.

Vicky

Health problems can also arise for other reasons:

My health generally is very good, but there is a tendency in a place like this, a bit like a school, for people to come in to visit with evil colds and flus. We send them home, because they shouldn't be here, but you do tend to pick up diseases. I've had about three colds in the last year, which is really unusual for me.

Jill

A lot of time I'm putting in heavy bits of equipment and carrying things around and it can be quite taxing. I do have back problems but that's a chronic thing, I just have to be very careful with what I do. If it flares up, the physiotherapist gives me ultrasound. It's just being aware of my limitations and knowing how to handle people and objects.

Occupational therapist

There may also be worries about health:

> When I first started out in this work, I used to think I had cancer a lot of the time. Any ache and pain and 'oh no, maybe I've got cancer'. Just working so closely with an illness that kills people, it's easy to take that on, because there are so many symptoms that could be something that you have yourself.
>
> *Michelle*

> I don't think this is a job you could do forever. You would burn out. You would lose your perspective on life that is living – you do become preoccupied by death. It is in my head a lot. You need to realise that there is other stuff going on out there, it is not just people coming in to die.
>
> *Claire*

There can also be an impact on emotional health:

> We all have moments where nothing's right. Like now, the staffing levels are low, we're very tired mentally and physically, people may be waking up and thinking they don't want to go to work – it's just that they are so tired. It can be depressing if you have a run of people who you don't feel you've managed well – they've died in pain or in distress. One or possibly two you expect, but any more than that, it does get to you – you start doubting yourself. You start questioning 'was it something I did or didn't do?'
>
> *Jessica*

> Sometimes you don't seem to have enough time in the day to do things that you should do. If you don't finish on time, you begin to question whether you've not managed your time properly. I always know when I need a holiday – the bags under my eyes become luggage. They seem to look extra long and heavy and my skin gets duller – you just know.
>
> *Nina*

This can occasionally be more serious:

> I suffered some depression not long ago. A friend said I was in mid-life transition – not mid-life crisis, but transition. And when you're feeling down, if you're not prepared to talk to anybody or acknowledge that you're feeling like that, you don't get anywhere. So people were very gently asking me if I was all right, knowing that I was someone who holds everything in.
>
> I also had some medical problems. The doctors thought I'd got an ulcer or something more sinister, which proved to be nothing as bad as it could have been. It never occurred to me how sinister it could be – my mind was

denying what was happening. I remember saying to a colleague, 'I've got a friend who's got all these symptoms, what would you recommend?' He said 'I would recommend to your friend that he sees his doctor as soon as possible. When are you going to make the appointment?'

Peter

Hospice work can also be so involving that family members are neglected:

I will probably look back and think over the years, I haven't given my family as much time as they should have had. Particularly my daughter – she had really bad post-natal depression and I really should have given her more time, I should have been more there for her. You need to be careful that you're not so busy caring for other people that you forget to care for those nearest to you.

Andrea

It affects the way that I relate to my family and my friends – when they're talking about their day, I really don't want to hear it, I've spent all day listening to other people. Sometimes I sit with my sister and I'm going 'yes, yes' and I'm not listening to what she's saying because I just want to switch off.

Vicky

My sons find it absolutely amazing that I can wash somebody's bottom, but under no circumstances could I wash an ashtray. And they want to know why I can be so sympathetic at work and everybody saying how lovely I am – and when I'm at home and they cut their finger off virtually to the bone, I say 'oh, wash it under the tap and put a plaster on it.' They say 'but you're meant to be a nurse'. I am, but I can't be sympathetic 24 hours a day.

Nina

In addition, friends may be ignored or new friendships not developed:

I live on my own. When I came to work at the hospice, I was just so enthusiastic and we were so short staffed that I gave it every minute I had. I lost contact with lots of friends – they kept saying 'we won't invite you because you can never come'. I've decided I'm not going to do that anymore. Friends are important.

Peter

I've moved 45 times in 47 years so developing and maintaining friendships for me has always been difficult. They seem very transitory. At the moment, I have two friends who are incredibly understanding of how little I see of them. When I spend up to ten hours of my day with people in lots of different contexts, I don't have a lot of energy for friends, and I feel a responsibility that I should.

Maggie

The combination of pressures can lead staff to consider quitting this line of work – sometimes frequently:

I have thought of quitting, many a time. You do get stressed, you have been told off maybe for something that's minor and you think, well, there is no need for that, and you want to hand in your resignation. We have people saying they are going to hand in their notice loads of times.

Dan

Sometimes, I just can't see another person – that's it, I'm not seeing any more today. I see the most difficult patients. They take a lot of thought on what's the right way to deal with them. It's hard to take it out of your head, because often the issues aren't resolved and you know you're going to go back the next day. How many times have any of us said 'I'm not going to carry on doing this!'

Consultant

Have I ever thought about leaving? Pretty much on a daily basis, but that's a recognition of the reason why I stay as well. I do rant and rave – there isn't a day goes by that I don't have a rant like 'this place is driving me crazy' and, that helps. If I say I am so frustrated or I'm kicking my filing cabinet yet again, I know that in doing that, I'm recognising that I can leave, I can go. But I'm also choosing not to – and that sort of empowers me to keep going. This type of work is obviously feeding me.

Maggie

CHAPTER 8

Ways of coping

Whatever the many difficulties and frustrations of hospice work, most people find ways of overcoming them to their own satisfaction. The issue of coping is not, however, straightforward. This chapter explores the many avenues available and some of the complexities involved.

Keeping work out of the home

Over and over, people insist that they try hard not to take work home with them:

> I'm quite good at being able to leave my work at work. You just have to make sure it stays here. As soon as I put my coat on to leave, I shut my folder, put it in my drawer and then things can wait until tomorrow. Obviously, there are some cases that do play on your mind – if someone's really unwell and you've been working with them for a long time, you wonder if that patient will be there tomorrow.
>
> *Charlotte*

> I taught myself years ago that I leave work at work – and home is home. You need that switch off. Once I put my clothes on, I'm back to me, I'm not the carer. One of my managers taught me – I used to worry about things, 'will this be done? will that be done?' and she said 'no, you leave it, it will be done, don't worry.'
>
> *Megan*

The fact that it is a *job* is stressed:

> At the end of the day, this is a job. I love it, but it's a job and when I leave work, that's my family life. You have to remember it's a job, because it will impact on your own life and once it impacts on your own life, it impacts back onto work. I have no intentions of leaving it, but it's a job.
>
> *Nina*

> It sounds awful, but I've learned to be very compassionate and supportive to the patients whilst I'm here, then I can leave it at the door. It's a job at the end of day – you're doing a job of work. If you took it home with you,

you'd be forever worrying about other people. You've got to look after your own family.

Laura

Some find special ways of helping them to leave work behind:

When I walk in the hospice, I put a cloak on – 'now I'm working in the hospice, I'm here to do my job'. And when I leave here, I take the cloak off – 'now I'm going out into the big world and I'm going to live my life'. It can affect your life. I can't change what's happening to people, I can just help the journey a little bit. It may seem harsh, but it's the only way you survive.

Andrea

For me, it's down to this uniform, keeping the boundaries, knowing when to function as a therapist or with another hat on elsewhere. My home is my sanctuary and I need that space, just the same as if I was stacking shelves in a shop. I wouldn't want the general public in my home, wondering about whether I charged them the right price for something. We all need our privacy.

Alice

But some do find that it can be difficult to forget work completely:

I'd like to think that I leave it behind when I go home, but nobody can do that 100%. You do have a little flash in your mind sometimes. You might see somebody that makes you think of something. But I don't purposefully carry things around in my mind. If I want to know about somebody's condition, I won't go home and look it up on the internet. I will speak to the appropriate staff here or see if there's something in the library, but I'll do it here.

Alice

I don't want to walk out of the door and forget the hospice 100%. That would mean I don't like what I'm doing. You should be able to have it with you, but not so that it dominates your life. Once or twice, I've had a sleepless night and the next day I've dashed in very early. That's one reason why I try to tie up loose ends before I go home at night. Each person has their own strategy for dealing with things like that.

Grace

Support from family and friends

Although many spouses and partners are said to be very supportive, there is a reluctance to impose hospice work on them:

I don't offload onto my husband in any great depth. He will ask what kind of a day I've had and I might say it was a bit grim. I told him the first time I saw a body in the mortuary, that kind of conversation. I don't feel it appropriate to talk to him about particular situations where there's real angst. I'd be disclosing details of people's lives that they've given to me in good faith.

Nicola

My husband is helpful and supportive. He knows what happens in here, but he doesn't want to hear the gory details and I don't need to tell him. I could sit him down and go through a catalogue of what I do in a day and he would need a whisky at the end of it. So I will have the whisky and he can just go to work! I don't think it would be fair – he doesn't bring his job home, I don't bring mine home.

Fiona

My husband and my sons are very supportive. On very odd occasions, something may play on my mind – probably around a relative and how I can help them cope or what we can do to make it easier. I'll try not to discuss it. You do have to protect your family. You have to be very careful because of confidentiality anyway.

Nina

There is a particular reluctance to impose anything on children:

I try to keep it contained. My daughter asked me only this week 'mum, do you see dead people?' and I said 'every week'. And she said 'do you touch them?' When I said yes, she said she didn't know – horror, horror! So you do contain it, because people find it awkward. This week, when I went home, I was quiet and my daughter wanted to go out and I said 'actually, I just need to be quiet, it has been quite a difficult day'. They know to leave it there and I don't need to do any more than that.

Claire

My adult son and I are really, really close, but he is not the sort of person that goes for the caring profession. He will listen – if he knows something is really bothering me, he will let me bounce off him. But he calls it the 'sad stories' – 'oh no, it is not the sad stories' kind of thing, so I tend not to tell him things.

Carole

Indeed, it is felt that children often do not really understand the work at all:

My children know I work in a hospice and a comment was made about wiping somebody's bum once – 'how can you do that all day?' I said 'do you think there are 50 people lined up with backsides out for me to wipe? It doesn't work like that!' But they don't need to know what I do. I tell them briefly, but you can see the lights go off – they are not interested, they want to listen to their music.

Fiona

Sometimes, other relatives may be a help:

I've got two sisters. One lives near me, so we see each other once a fortnight or so, but we're often chatting on the phone once a week. She's very supportive. Protective as well. She'll try and resolve issues for me, because when we were children she would always sort my problems out. Apparently I didn't have to say anything for a couple of years, because she did all the talking, 'What's your name?' 'His name's Peter.' 'How old are you?' 'He's two and a half.'

Peter

Good friends can prove important here:

It's necessary to make time to be with good friends, people who you can be totally honest with, when you have something that you're not feeling too happy about. A good friend where you can just say 'I've had a crap day' and them just being there is enough. We all need a good mate.

Alice

There's friends and there's friends. There are some people where you can say what you like to and they don't take it personally. They know when to pull away and say 'it's good he's shared that with me, it's not going to be spoken about'. I've got one friend, where we both know what we tell each other no one else will hear about. That's really helpful to know, but I don't burden them.

Peter

Often, these work in similar professions:

I have friends who work in hospitals and sometimes we get together and it's easier. We don't always talk about work, but if you say you've had an awful day, they know exactly what you're talking about. Sometimes we end up talking if there has been a difficult case – not moaning, but just letting off the steam.

Julia

Most of my friends are medical, people who I've trained with, but we don't talk medicine all the time. We talk about all sorts of other things. I never talk much about this work with people. I think it's a private sort of thing – it's people's lives that you've been privileged enough to be part of right at the end.

Consultant

But some friends can find it hard to understand what goes on in a hospice and do not, in fact, really want to know:

Some friends understand about my work and some don't. I have friends who talk about their work and when I talk about mine, they tend to say 'can we change the subject, please?'

Dan

I live with a number of others in a house share – they're all business people, office people, with no comprehension of what my day-to-day work is like. I wouldn't talk to them about what I do at work.

Rebecca

Most of my friends are not medical and I think they find it bizarre that I chose this specialty, when you imagine that as a doctor, you're going to cure people. Some of my friends haven't seen anyone die, so for me to say I have seen many people die, they just can't fathom it.

Doctor 1

And there is a need to get away from work completely:

With some friends, if you're not careful, all you'll talk about is what's happening at work. And I'm thinking 'don't ask me about that, let's get away from work'. If you're not careful, it's 24/7.

Peter

I don't have a wide circle of friends. I don't have a major social life. I do the things that I want to do and I just find I don't need it. When I'm not working, I don't want to see anybody. Some people say that's really unsociable, but I just find at the end of the day, when you've just had constant contact with people like we do, I don't really want it – I want to get away from people.

William

There is also a sense that their priorities have made them somewhat apart from others:

Sometimes I finish work and get on the train and I just think none of these people have any idea what I've had to do today, what I've had to say today, what I've experienced. People have no idea when they say 'oh I've had such a hard day'. You think, have you really? It's all part of doing our job, but it is very hard.

Rebecca

If I worked in Sainsbury's, I would be worrying about mundane rubbish in my life. Certainly, in this job, you don't worry about the mundane stuff. You go home and if your friends are moaning about their bills or the state of their hair, you think 'get life into perspective, you are not bloody dying'.

Diana

Once, I went home and somebody had kicked our car outside my home and my husband was very distraught. I said 'I'm sorry I can't get too worked up about it, we've just had a 31-year-old woman admitted today, so somebody kicking the car, it doesn't mean anything to me'.

Louise

Finding ways to relax

Like people in any job, people working in hospices have varying ways of relaxing. Some stress that they will ignore housework if they need to relax:

If the windows need cleaning and I don't feel like doing it, I don't do it. I think it's not going to benefit me to do that. I have to pace myself. Will another day make that much difference to the windows, if I would benefit more from what I call – it's a Danish term – *schlumeking*. A *schlumek* is one of those days where you put your old tracksuit on and read a magazine and think oh, never mind.

Alice

I try not to do too much at home. If I feel tired, if I have had some particularly stressful days in here, the next day I am not going to think I've got to get up and hoover. Working here has taught me you don't worry about things like that, the sky is not going to fall down because I don't run the hoover round. So I have an easy day – I just think it will wait and it does.

Fiona

Some do things with their family:

My partner and I laugh a lot and we watch a lot of comedy on TV. He's incredibly understanding of the fact that every single job I do, I will always put more into it than other people do, or think I should. He knows I'm happiest when I'm able to be creative.

Maggie

One of my children just had a baby recently. Last night, I just thought I haven't seen this child for a week and I phoned her up this morning and said 'put the kettle on I am coming round, I need to hug that boy.' So I had a big hug before I came to work – he is so gorgeous. My children are very, very important to me.

Claire

Some undertake very physical activities:

I go to the park or roller-blading with friends. I try to go to the gym or go running – that's quite a good release, even if you think about things while you're doing it. I do feel better after that.

Charlotte

There have been times when I've gone home feeling really sad and wanting to cry. I live opposite a park and I go for a little walk in the park and rant and rave to God, or dig the garden and see if there's any new life coming up in the garden. I manage it that way.

Nicola

I run. I have always been fairly physically active all my life. I started running marathons two or three years ago. I go out in the evenings and run five miles – that's a great way to clear your brain. You do think when you're running, you go over some things you've dealt with during the day. I find it extremely therapeutic.

William

There are also cultural outlets:

When I get home, I have a nice hot bath and just relax. I won't go out drinking and all that. I sing in a choir, which is one big thing that helps me with my stress.

Dan

I work only four days a week, so I have long weekends when I do painting, something completely different. It is only a hobby, watercolours – portraits.

Diana

I have all sorts of outside interests. I play instruments and we do a lot of artistic things. I garden. You need diversions from this work. It is very intense at times and you need to get away. But I don't let it interfere with my enjoyment of life.

William

And some mainly relax with friends or colleagues:

> I've got friends who I socialise with and we'll go for drinks or go for a meal. I've made a decision since I've been back from holiday to get away on short breaks, so I've been doing that.
>
> *Ken*

> When the hospice staff go out together, we get up to what everybody else gets up to! We might go to a restaurant, we can behave quite badly. Everybody knows how to have a really good time. We go out to dinner and we drink too much, we have fun, we have a lot of laughs.
>
> *Louise*

Support from the hospice

Hospice managers tend to be aware of needs for support and offer various avenues to assist staff. Some have meetings built into the system, either on a regular or ad hoc basis:

> There are bereavement sessions, which are very good. You go through everyone who's died since the last meeting – who was on duty, was it a good death, did we achieve our aims, do the social workers need to follow up and so forth. If you don't get to that meeting, then you miss it until the next time. It's a while since I've been to one.
>
> *Helen*

> We encourage people to 'debrief', if necessary. We had a debriefing recently after a young woman died. Basically, we set a time for those people who might want to come together and chat for an hour. We had two or three doctors there and staff who weren't even on duty that day. Our consultant put things into perspective, saying that this woman did have a very advanced disease, so it was not really surprising that she died. We have done this a few times, but not really often.
>
> *Eileen*

Or there can be more informal arrangements for support:

> When I'm running the shift, about 11.30–12.00 in the morning, I will make a cup of tea for the whole staff, call them into the office – and I will do that again at 4.00. I sit them down – obviously if someone buzzes, that will be answered – but it's a case of 'right, sit down, have a cup of tea'. And you will just chit-chat, but you know that if you're finding something a bit stressful or if you've got something on your mind, there is always someone that you can go to and get it off your chest.
>
> *Sister*

At lunchtime, we have what we call 'protected time' where you can say what you like and no one's going to take offence. Within reason, of course. The nurses are sometimes in very intense situations, where they'll want to laugh, but can't. They've mopped up a lot of stress, a lot of emotions, and they need to let it off somehow. So we have that policy where if you want to say something to me at lunchtime, I'm not going to take it personally. If you lose your rag, that's good – you've lost it with me and not with a patient.

Head of hospice 2

Some professions within a hospice have a tradition of regular supervision, whether formal or informal:

I have a clinical supervisor and she gives me a lot of reassurance. Working as a sole occupational therapist, it's been quite challenging. It's very useful having a supervisor – just to bounce ideas off her and to realise that she also experiences some of the things I do.

Occupational therapist

Once every six weeks, we have a therapists meeting where we start off with a chance for supervision, if we need to discuss anything that's happened. We go over things in general, anything that's bothering us, anything that is not working or whatever. It's a chance to offload, so you don't take things home.

Complementary therapist

Supervision is always available, but I've been a bit unwilling to face it. I thought chaplains don't ask about supervision, we deal with these things ourselves. We're not good in the Church at recognising what we need.

Chaplain 3

Counselling of various kinds may also be available:

We counsel staff and volunteers, if they need it. New members of staff will often experience thoughts of their own mortality, in all sorts of ways – 'I don't feel well, am I going to die of cancer?' You can become quite obsessed with death and you need to find ways of coping with that.

If someone needs a lot of sessions, I've got one particular counsellor I send them to. If they want just one or two sessions, I do that. But if there's events happening in their own life, I send them to somebody else, because ethically it's not good that I see them. You want somebody to feel free to say anything, not thinking they're going to meet me next week on the wards.

Counsellor 2

Over the years, a lot of people have asked me for individual support and I have to be careful that they feel comfortable afterwards. People wouldn't always want to share their most personal feelings, particularly when they've got to work with somebody the next day.

Social worker

And staff often talk to each other informally:

This is a beautiful place to work in. I know that I can get support from anybody, from the lowest to the highest level. Everybody makes you feel that you can come and talk to them, so you don't feel alone. If you're stressed, even if you don't say so, somebody usually picks it up and says 'you need to slow down'.

Grace

I've got peer support from the other lead nurses. It's a very open organisation, so if I have a problem I can go to anybody. I can go to the head of the hospice and say 'can I get a cup of coffee, I need a chat', without having to make an appointment. Everybody can access such support.

Head nurse

Thank God, it is a great team. You are very much reliant on offloading on colleagues. If we have had a particularly bad week or if a young patient that we have known has died, we will go to the pub or for a meal and offload on each other.

Diana

The support you get is fantastic. When my mum died, I even had volunteers coming up to me saying 'I'm really sorry, do let me know if there's anything I can do' – it ranged from them right up to the head of the hospice. On the other side, everyone knows everything about everyone. It's like living in a village, but when the chips are down, they're all there for you.

Jessica

But sometimes there is a wish for more support:

I'd like a time set aside to actually discuss difficult situations, whether it be a patient dying or their treatment or the family. We have a lot of difficult patients, but we don't have a proper set time to discuss it. This job is tremendously draining emotionally, especially where you can get three or four deaths in one night. It's really important that you're given the opportunity to talk – and the time.

Vicky

We're supposed to have reflective meetings once a week to discuss particular patients – a kind of case conference about care around a patient that maybe we weren't all in agreement with. We were doing those weekly, but that has stopped – people have been too busy.

Michelle

There's not really anybody for me to talk to. One of the other doctors and I will talk and that can be helpful, but doctors are very poor at providing moral and psychological support to each other. They feel they have to be independent and manage their own psychological health.

Consultant

Own spirituality

Another source of support is a person's religion or spiritual beliefs:

I am a Catholic. I still question things and I'm not here to convert people. I do think it helps me to try not to be selfish and to have some kind of goodness, to do the best for people. There's something there that's better than what people are experiencing in life. When I worked in intensive care, you'd find things like a baby who got run over by a milk float and you wonder why things like that happen. Having a belief in the afterlife definitely helps me.

Catherine

I'm a Christian – I believe that Jesus is the Way, the Truth and the Life. And that when we die, the Lord Jesus Christ will give judgment on everybody. The best I can do for my patients is pray for them. I'm not asked to do so very often, but occasionally one will ask. I believe very much in God's ability to heal. Everything is in His hands. We're pilgrims on this earth – here for a purpose, and when we get to heaven, we will give account to God. For me, it makes working here easier – this is what God prepared me to do.

Grace

I'm attracted to aspects of Buddhism and the principles of living your life with loving kindness and heartfulness. I love the phrase 'walk gently, but carry a big stick'. But for me probably, it's the heartfulness and paying attention to what is in the moment. The phrase 'this, too, will pass' I find really helpful.

Maggie

But not everyone has this form of solace:

Quite a lot of professionals who go into palliative care are religious and I sort of envy them that – maybe it makes a bit more sense of what we see. If I had strong religious beliefs that patients were going to a better place, it would make it much easier. I don't have any belief, so it all seems a kind of mockery.

Diana

I don't have a faith. I don't really know what keeps me going. I believe your life is planned out for you, so you've just got to follow that journey and whatever happens, happens. Maybe I've been put here to help those who need that support through that journey.

Vicky

I was brought up singing in the church choir, but I've never kept it going on a regular basis. I have a bit of a jaundiced view and I don't bring religion at all into what I do. I love some of the rituals – we've lost a lot of the rituals around death. It's an expanding area in palliative care, but I'm not judgemental in any way.

William

Working in a hospice can make people question their beliefs, especially when they see people dying early or under difficult circumstances:

You do get your faith shaken. Why would someone have cancer and then a heart attack and then a stroke? Some people have everything happen to them and you just think, why? Or if a patient's got young children or they've just got married, I think it's really unfair. You try to justify things, but at the end of the day, that's life. There's a lot of suffering in the world and we just need to do the best that we can.

Charlotte

I was brought up a Catholic. I don't practise now, but I do believe in a life after death. But my beliefs didn't help when one young patient died. When they're older, they've had their life, they've seen their grandchildren, sometimes their great-grandchildren and it is time for them to go, whereas with that one, she didn't even see her children grow up. It seems unfair.

Megan

But some have their faith strengthened:

I've always believed that there is a God or whatever you want to call it. And working here in the hospice, it has kind of confirmed that there must be something else there, because of seeing deaths and how peaceful people look afterwards.

Julia

I was brought up as a Catholic, but I don't go to services and things. But I am quite a spiritual person. I do believe there is something else when we go – because the amount of love that I see here between people is just too big to disappear when somebody dies. When you are with somebody all your life, that love is there and when somebody dies, it has got to go somewhere. Maybe that's how I get through the thought of dying. I would like to think that I will meet up with everybody and it is going to be a big hoolie upstairs, but I don't know.

Fiona

PART III

MOTIVATIONS AND REWARDS

CHAPTER 9

Initial motivation

One of the key questions for hospice staff is why do they undertake such work. But this breaks down into two issues: what brought them to the work in the first place and what rewards they gain from it once they are there. This chapter addresses the former, while the following one explores the latter.

A sense of vocation

Some people might imagine that people who choose to work in a hospice have a long-standing sense of vocation. And, indeed, there are some people who have always known what they wanted to do with their lives:

> I always wanted to be a nurse and throughout my training I always knew I wanted to work with cancer. Obviously, here we do more than just cancer, but I always wanted to look after the dying.
>
> *Rebecca*

> I have always been drawn to bereavement. All the time at college, I kept saying I wanted to work with bereavement and everybody kept asking why. I said 'well, life is a bereavement'. Life is a series of losses, really – marriages break up, opportunities are lost – it is not just death. It is just an area I have been drawn to. I don't know why.
>
> *Claire*

Some are prompted to work in a hospice by a particular experience with one:

> I've done shop work, I've worked in a café, I've done child-minding – you name it, I've done it. But I had always wanted to be a nurse and I always knew that I wanted to do palliative care. Halfway through my training, my dad died in a hospice and I saw the care that he got and it was 'I want to do that'. Working in hospitals, you just can't give the care you were trained for. As a staff nurse, you're just doing pen pushing. So I knew that I wanted to work in a hospice.
>
> *Jessica*

> My mum died at a hospice when I was in my early twenties. I was really impressed with the standard of care. I just knew that that was

something I wanted to get into – it was the intimacy, the openness
between the staff and the family. We were very well informed and we
were all looked after holistically – it was something that I hadn't been
exposed to before. I'd always been quite alarmed in hospitals that
people who were dying were still being tested for various things, they
were on their own, their families weren't informed, there was no
privacy.

Michelle

After having three babies, I decided that I needed to get my brain working
again and did an Open University course, Care in the Community. One of
the modules was about people dying. I spent a morning here and I remember thinking 'I like the feel of this place'. I went about my work for about
a year, but kept thinking about the hospice and I rang one day to ask if
there was a possibility of a job. It took 18 months, because when people
come here, they seem to stay.

Fiona

And some may be responding to their experience of working in other settings:

I worked on an acute medical ward, looking after nine patients, which is
normal for a staff nurse in the NHS. But you can't look after nine patients
properly – people are actually not getting the treatment they need. I
wanted to give the best that I could. I wanted somewhere where staff
nurses had a good ratio to patients. Here, you're not as stressed, you know
that you've got time. Some patients can take between an hour and a half to
two hours to get washed fully, but you know you've got the time to do that.
At the end of a day, you can finish work knowing that you have given the
best you can for that patient.

Helen

I spent a number of years at a hospital doing oncology nursing and
reached a stage where I needed a different challenge. I wanted to stay in
the area of cancer and the opportunity came up for a community palliative
care nurse, so I applied for that. It meant a change from the hospital environment to community, as well as being more focused on palliative care,
rather than administering treatments. The focus on death and dying
wasn't something that made me want to come into it – it was just an
opportunity to do something different.

Community nurse

I was a senior nurse in the NHS. I was working in education, helping staff,
and although it was fascinating, I didn't really have any impact on people
and patients. I wanted to do something a bit more worthwhile. I had
worked in an intensive care unit – it's not uncommon for intensive care

nurses to go to hospices – you are used to talking to relatives about the potential of a death and what to do after a death.

Catherine

Prior experience of death

Other experiences can be formative toward working with dying people. A key one is personal experience of illness or death and dying:

> A defining moment for me would be when my father committed suicide. I saw an advert to train as a bereavement counsellor and I thought what a brilliant idea, I would have liked to have had bereavement counselling. It was very good training, a very high standard – I really enjoyed it and discovered that I was quite good at it. But I then decided to go back and finish off my social work training. I saw an ad some time later for a job caring for people with terminal illnesses – I thought that would be interesting and applied. I think it's partly because of my father, that's really how I started to think about death and dying in a much more coherent way.
>
> *Social worker*

> My mum had a mini stroke and I looked after her. My aunt said 'you should do this for a living' and I thought I'd try it. I'd heard of it because a lot of my social services clients came here for respite or to die. I didn't know how I would handle the death bit. I just rang and asked them if they had any vacancies and as luck had it, they did. I wished I'd come here a long time ago.
>
> *Megan*

There may be something significant about having a lot of bereavements in the family:

> My brother and sister-in-law died within a short time of each other. That was probably the driving force. It wasn't so much their deaths, it was more the fact that there wasn't much support – I wanted to redress that somehow. I can also remember my grandfather dying at home, when I was only five. He had throat cancer and I can distinctly remember the noise of his voice when I went to say goodbye to him.
>
> *Andrea*

> My father died of a heart attack and a couple of years later my brother-in-law died of cancer. So I brought those two experiences to it. Initially, each time I walked down the drive here, my stomach would turn in knots, until I realised that being alongside people was not simply what I could give, but that I needed also to receive. I felt very emotionally drained when I came away from a patient – perhaps I was identifying the person with my father.

Then I thought if I'm going to do this, to be alongside others, I need to be able to step away or deal with my own issues.

Nicola

I lost my mother when I was only 22. My father moved abroad and I was left with my grandmother who had some sort of dementia. And then my father died and then his aunt died and then my grandmother died, one a year. We were a very small family, so at about 40, I was the matriarch of my family. Perhaps it gave me an understanding of what it is like to be without the people you need in your life.

Claire

Seeing poor care of relatives at the time of their deaths can also provide a strong incentive to offer something better:

A lot of people end up in their medical specialties because of things that happened in their life. When my father was dying of cancer, nobody paid attention to details like the fact he was up all night in pain. And nobody could advise on appropriate painkillers and, when he was given some, they were inadequate. That wouldn't have changed his outcome, but my mother's memory was very much that he suffered. So it wasn't him dying, it was what led up to his death that could have changed. The fact that no doctors or nurses paid attention to detail had a big impact on me.

Doctor 1

I'm an Irish Catholic and it's a tradition to go to funerals of family and friends and even people you didn't know. My mum would take us to attend the Mass of an old lady or old man whose name she knew and she knew there wouldn't be anybody there – she felt that was very important. In some ways, it probably goes back as far as that. But it wasn't until later that I started losing aunts and uncles and my dad died – that it started hitting home. I suppose this affected my interest in palliative care.

One uncle, who died in hospital in the mid-1970s, had cancer. He was in Ireland and there wasn't palliative care as such. The symptoms were badly controlled. He had a lot of pain and he had people trooping in and out to visit him, when they should have been gently told that it wasn't appropriate. The whole thing was badly managed in many ways. Hospital, where everything is buzzing around about you, is not a conducive place for someone who wants to die peacefully – you need a peaceful environment.

Eileen

Even seeing poor care in a professional capacity can have a large impact:

I was trained in medicine here in the UK, but I worked abroad for many years. I trained as a general physician. When the so-called 'AIDS epidemic' hit us in the early 1980s, I got rather involved looking after these people really by default, because none of my physician colleagues were terribly interested. There was very little we could do with them, other than try to keep them comfortable and manage their death. Of course, AIDS is quite a different disease now, but that's how I got into it.

I was not very happy at the way my consultant colleagues looked after their dying patients. It was the old story – the dying people in a general hospital were relatively ignored once they were reaching the terminal phase. People were afraid to go in and talk to them and symptom management was very rudimentary. I was quite upset about that. So it just stemmed from there. I eventually moved from one hospital to another, where they allowed me to develop a palliative care unit.

Consultant

Other formative experiences

But there are other kinds of experiences which may affect a person's motivation to help others. Some trace the roots of their interest in serving others to formative experiences in their childhood:

I grew up in Northern Ireland during the height of 'the troubles'. At any given moment, you could be in great danger. You can't help but have that form you in some way or other, whether you're conscious of it or not. Death and dying was pretty much what you thought about a lot. It was around.

Once, my friend and I were at the theatre and had to leave early to catch the last bus home. We were walking down the street when there was an explosion about four streets away – the IRA had just blown up the gas works. We heard soldiers running down the road shouting – one of them picked me up, another one picked my friend up, and threw us over a hedge into someone's front garden. Armoured jeeps came squealing down the road behind them. We just sat behind the hedge and talked about the play until we were allowed to continue on – we missed the bus and ended up walking the four miles home. Another time, I was on a bus and a bomb was actually on the bus – we got off and stood at the other end of the street and waited for the bus to be blown up and then we walked up the street and got back on another bus and went home. I didn't get home till 10.00 that night and, when I came in, Mum said 'your dinner's in the oven' – we didn't talk about what happened, because these were everyday occurrences.

Maggie

When I was seven, I got TB-sinuvitis and spent two years in hospital at Margate. There were no cures in those days for TB – I spent six months on my back with a weight on my leg because my knee was beginning to

crush. I was there, seven years of age, taken away from my family for the first time and then suddenly being served breakfast. I said 'what's that?' and the nurse said, 'that's bacon', and I said 'I can't eat bacon.' The sister came towards me – I can still see her in front of me in the old blue, crisp, starched uniform – and said 'now what's all this nonsense about you not eating bacon?' I said 'I can't, if I eat bacon, God will strike me down dead'. She said 'why?' I said 'because I'm Jewish' and she said 'I've never heard such nonsense – eat it!' And I ate it. That experience just made me, somewhere in the back of my mind. We were looked after wonderfully.

My father arrived in this country at the age of 14, in charge of four younger siblings. He instilled in all of us the love of the country, because the country had taken him in, it had given him an opportunity. He was very, very proud of the time he was naturalised – or as he called it 'nationalised'. He instilled in all of us that we must be proud of being British and give back something to the community. It is gratitude for allowing us to be here. Despite the fact that he didn't have very much, money was always given to charity. He also tried to look after relatives, who were in a much worse situation than he was. The Jewish culture teaches you that you must give back.

Volunteer 1

When I was at school, you were given either old people's gardens to look after or autistic kids of the same kind of age – I went straight to the autistic kids. Great work. And both my mum and my grandma did volunteering. In the 1970s, my mum used to abandon her three children to her husband for two months every year and go look after lepers. So it really is there. I come from a huge family, we're very close and I lost a lot of very close family members in a short space of time, from my mid-teens to mid-20s. So as I continued to volunteer, I tended to be drawn towards that sort of thing. When you go through some tough family times when you're very young, you learn an awful lot about grieving, so it can be a great way to put something back.

Volunteer coordinator

The accidental route

But the number of people who wind up working in a hospice almost by accident is surprising:

I was working in a hospital and was phoned up by a company who were recruiting people working in oncology to go for an interview at the hospice. They must have got me on a really bad day and I agreed to have a look. I didn't really know what to expect, but I thought it would be dull, gloomy and depressing. I was really pleasantly surprised – the place was bright and the staff were friendly and happy. It was very different from an

NHS ward and I thought wow, it's really nice. I was very eager to come for a follow up interview and it all went very quickly and I accepted the job.

Charlotte

I came here really quite by accident. My actual training is art school – I did graphic design. But then I had a family and things changed and I had a job in a family planning clinic. I quite liked the medical world. I lived fairly near here and there was an advert in the local paper for part-time people.

Louise

I started very young as a journalist and then worked in public relations of various kinds. At some point, I thought I'm turning middle aged and I don't want this kind of job anymore – and by sheer chance I saw this job advertised. I was delighted because I knew what the place had done over the years as I live nearby. It landed on my lap at the right time. I can't say I had a particular interest in palliative care. I'd volunteered for about 20 years in all kinds of areas and worked very closely with nurses, for instance, taking severely disabled people on holiday.

Volunteer coordinator

My original career was in finance, but through the years I had also done some caring jobs – going out and putting people to bed, doing meals and that type of thing. People always used to say that I should become a counsellor, because I listened to people. And I kept thinking yes, it was something I would do one of these days. Then a friend signed up for a counselling course and encouraged me to go, too. I got a placement here in the day hospice and then later on, they were looking for volunteer counsellors. And that's how I started.

Counsellor 2

CHAPTER 10

What makes the work worthwhile

By whatever route staff come to work in a hospice, they tend to stay. There seem to be many reasons for their willingness – or, indeed, eagerness – to do so.

Feeling involved

The rewards of working in a hospice are expressed in many different ways. Over and over, people speak of loving their work:

> Sometimes people ask me how I can do this job. I say I do it because I love it. I would never do anything else. I love it and I know I'm good at it from the response of patients and their relatives and my colleagues. I think I shouldn't waste whatever it is I've got to be able to look after people who are dying. There is such satisfaction in being able to give someone a good death.
>
> *Rebecca*

> I absolutely love what I do. Not many people can say that. It can be sad at times, of course, but in general this is a very happy place. I'm not a do-gooder, not 'dedicating my life'. We're just like everybody else – good, bad and awful. But it's a great honour to be allowed to be involved in other people's lives, which includes their deaths.
>
> *Louise*

Perhaps the most common single word that people use is that it is a 'privilege' to be there:

> It is truly amazing to be involved in people's lives when they are so vulnerable. It is a privilege to be allowed to be involved in that part of their life, when they are raw and exposed. Two weeks ago, the father of a good friend was here and died. I was quite involved with the family right to the end. People allow you in, they are very trusting and that trust is quite humbling. I almost felt I needed to write my friend a letter to thank her for allowing me to be part of it, because that's how it left me feeling. How amazing to be able to be of some help.
>
> *Claire*

I'm a carer by nature. The hospice seems to be an environment that I'm suited to. It is the privilege of sharing time, very precious time – being in close proximity with people when they feel their time on earth is limited. You may be the person that they may tell something to, just 'oh, I never realised how beautiful a sunset was'. You may be privileged to hear something that is so special to that individual, that can be an awakening for them. You should feel very privileged for that.

Alice

When we go through our own lives, usually we wouldn't dream of impinging on other people's lives unless we're a friend or a relative. Now, for someone to allow me to be at this stage of their life, to take me as I am and to allow me to help them is a privilege. We wouldn't entertain someone just dropping in to such an important part of our life, unless we trusted them. And if people trust us to be part of their life, then that is a privilege.

Eileen

Part of this is the one-to-one contact, with sufficient time for it to feel personal:

The best thing is being able to have hands-on contact with patients, like giving a patient a bed bath. It takes me back to why I wanted to be a nurse, which was to have that personal input, rather than just doing a load of paperwork. It's one-on-one care. If nurses knew before what they know after their training, many would probably have gone to be healthcare assistants. They are doing what we want to do, the personal care side of things.

Sister

When I worked in a hospital, I didn't have as much patient contact. I would see someone once and then do loads of paperwork and refer them on to someone else. Now, I follow someone through their whole journey – I'm involved with them from the moment they get referred until they either get discharged or they pass away. It's probably one of the best decisions that I could have made to come work here.

Occupational therapist

There is also deep satisfaction in making a contribution to others:

It does give you joy to feel that you are alleviating mental and emotional suffering. I can't do anything about their physical suffering, but I can be there if they want a priest. It's a bit of a cliché, but often the nursing staff will say they get more from the patient than they give – it's true. I am inspired by them. I'm not a patient man myself and I think how on earth do some of them cope so readily?

Chaplain 1

I like the fact that, in a small way, you can maybe make a difference to people's lives and relatives' memories of them. It is a vocation working in a hospice. You have to want to do it and get some satisfaction out of it. It is not rocket science, it is just attention to detail. If you can change someone's focus, so they are not totally absorbed with pain – they can't sleep, they are crying, they want to end their life – to someone who is pain free and going home for a period of time, that's fantastic.

Doctor 1

Responding to challenges

Some clearly like the challenges entailed by the work. For instance, it can be tricky to find the right way of controlling pain and other symptoms:

I love symptom control. If a patient has come in with pain or nausea, it's trying to get on top of those things and making their quality of life better. Two people with nausea might have totally different causes. And you never know what's going to happen in the next hour – it's constantly being aware and adapting to what's going on through the periods of the day.

Jessica

It's a fascinating line of work. I've done other sorts of medicine, but in a truly humanistic way, you really feel you do achieve something. And every person with a life threatening illness presents a new challenge. They're never the same. It's addicting doing this work.

I have to prioritise, so I end up by seeing the more difficult ones, the ones with complex pain. Lots of psychological angst that manifests itself in physical symptoms. That's an area that I find fascinating. I see people who are getting buckets of drugs and nothing works – and you know that this is a more psychological angst. It's a challenge to try to work through that, because you know and they know the drugs are not the issue. But there's nothing more satisfying than working someone around, whose pain ends up being well controlled on a minimal amount of drugs, because you've dealt with the underlying psychological and existential issues.

Consultant

But others also find other challenges, such as encouraging patients to eat:

I like coming to work and thinking 'what can I do to make this person's quality of life better?' And because it could be a patient's last meal, the hospice is very good at allowing you a decent budget. And because the portions are small, you can make nice things.

It's challenging trying to get enough calories in the food, so that people can eat a very small portion, but it has some calorific value. A lot of drugs make things taste salty, so we thought we cannot put salt in, so how do we get flavour? Let's buy parsley, coriander and mint – we use lots of herbs, spice. It was a learning curve. Get a good greengrocer and good companies to supply fresh meat, make fresh soups every day. Some patients haven't tasted food for weeks and weeks – if you don't taste food, you are not going to eat it.

Some of the high calorie drinks taste vile, but you can tart them up by putting ice-cream and ice-cubes in them. We put bananas in them, so they are getting extra potassium. It also helps to get people to drink it through a straw. I explain to patients that there are 600 calories in one of them, so if you can substitute that for a little bit of food, you are putting quite a lot of calories in. Their energy levels go up a little bit and that's what my aim is – to make people stay awake, rather than getting into a coma-like state. I tell them 'I am sure you want to spend the next two or three weeks with your family, reminiscing and saying all the things you want to say'.

I have never once woken up and thought I don't want to go to work. The day I feel like that is the day I start looking for other employment.

Chef

Another challenge arises around finding a way through to help patients in denial:

I can remember one lady who was only about 30 and the whole thing was, 'I'm going to get better, I'm going to go home'. Even with the hints we'd dropped, she hadn't picked up that actually this was terminal. Her partner said to me 'I really need to talk to her and she's just not listening' and he said he really wanted me to tell her that she's dying. So we had that conversation and lots of tears, but at the end of it, it was 'thank you for telling me, because actually I've got a lot I want to do'. She didn't leave the hospice again, but she did everything that she wanted to do, all from her bed.

I couldn't change the fact that she was going to die. What you can do is make the journey easier for the patient and for their family – if you can do that, you've done the job, really.

Andrea

I had one patient who was in a room where you could see all the flowers outside. She wasn't saying much and we tried to get her to open up one day. It was sunny and the flowers looked really nice, so I asked if she could see the crocuses. And then I said 'after the crocuses…' I was about to say 'after they die', but I had to hold back – I said 'after the crocuses, we have daffodils and the grass is literally covered in yellow'. She said 'I won't see those – I won't be here'. I realised then that she knew she was dying. I just carried on talking with her. We had been trying for ages to get her to accept it.

Dan

Or it can be finding a way of helping people to die with greater peace:

> There was one patient, where I knocked on her door and introduced myself as the chaplain. She looked at me and said 'I've got nothing to say, but if you want to sit down, you can'. I sat down and 45 minutes later I left the room. She spoke for the whole time. She had a lot to say, but she had to ask me a few questions first, before she realised that she could talk to me. I prayed with her. And she was in tears, because she had found somebody who she felt she could talk to about her faith. I went back a few days later and she opened up and told me lots of things.
>
> When she died, the daughter said 'whatever you said to her that night, it changed her, she's now at peace'. And I thought wow, there's a lady who needed to talk and I made the opportunity. The Holy Spirit directed the conversation and she died a peaceful lady. So that was a wonderful experience of just being in the right place at the right time. I felt very humble that I was the vehicle for that.
>
> *Chaplain 2*

> I was with a terrible situation yesterday at someone's house. A father was dying not a great death at all and the family were refusing a lot of help. The dad was dying from alcoholic cirrhosis of the liver – he was supposed to get a transplant and never made it. A very angry son gave me an awful rant about the care his father had had over the last while. After I had just absorbed it all, he asked 'why the hell do you do this job? It must be awful,' and I replied 'well, somebody has to sort out people like you and deal with this situation with your father dying'. We talked a lot more and they were very grateful when I left.
>
> I went back this morning – the father's dying, he's very peaceful, he's comfortable, the family are all happy, sitting round the bed, not wanting any nurses or anybody. It's very satisfying. Even the ex-wife was there. That scenario was not what I walked into the day before. Yes, it's terribly sad and depressing at times, but there's such huge rewards when things go right. To turn what was a terrible, stressful, sad situation into something that is more memorable in a very positive way.
>
> *Consultant*

The variety of people

Much of hospice work involves working with a great variety of people. Some note the pleasures of meeting people of all kinds:

> The day care centre is my family. We've got some wonderful patients. One difficulty is that when you meet people for the first time, somewhere at the back of your mind, you wonder how long you're going to know them. But some of our patients do fine and live longer than expected. One old chap

said 'I'm going to stay around as long as I possibly can, just to prove that they're wrong!' If I'm away, I keep in touch. My life has been made richer by the people I've met here.

Volunteer 1

Part of this is the sense of shared experiences:

Our reflexologist told me how she came out of a session and saw a group of women sitting around a table – they were doing cross-stitching and chatting. She stood watching these women talking and sharing experiences, laughing, taking comfort in each other's company. It was that archetypal image of people sharing something really, really important, but really simple. For me palliative care is not just about helping people manage their suffering – it's about all these wonderful moments when they forget that they're in that state of suffering.

Day centre manager

And some speak of the intimacy involved in such encounters:

I have had some really profound conversations with people at night, when it has been quiet. That is where I feel I am really utilised. In other kinds of nursing, you don't have the time to do that. There is no pretence at this time, people are open about what is happening. They talk about the lives they've had, how they might do things differently if they had it over. A lot of stuff comes up. People feel they have learned something along the way and they want to share that with you before they go.

Michelle

I can't think of anything more wonderful than somebody saying thank you for something that you've done which you enjoyed doing. I can't think of anything more wonderful than walking into the day centre and feeling that sense of comfort in people spending time together, especially when I hear laughter. I can't think of anything more wonderful than the idea that if you care about someone, it matters. You never know what else could happen as a result of you caring – letting people touch your heart.

I like being in the moment with someone, whatever that moment might be, where nothing else matters. You don't protect it, you just pay attention to it, because the moments pass. Someone came to see me this morning just to tell me that she was feeling really bad today. All I needed to do was just acknowledge it with her. She chose to come to the centre when she was feeling bad, which was what was important.

Day centre manager

And part of the variety of people is remembering particular patients. Only a few can be noted here. Some are remembered for their age:

One patient is quite raw in my mind – a young girl. I did a lot of her care, so I spent a lot of time with her, we used to have a giggle together and became very close. She was here for six weeks. And she just suddenly died. On the Saturday, I said 'I'll see you Monday'– and when I came in, she was dead. We were all knocked sideways by it. She was younger than me.

You try to keep your distance, but you can't help it, because you do a long shift, you do become involved. You get to know all the family and everyone who comes in visiting. You can't help but get close. If she was upset, I would sit with her and chat and then we would end up laughing and I knew she was OK. She was such a jolly person. Some people keep their distance, but she wasn't like that – if she wanted a hug, you'd give her a hug.

Megan

The patient that sticks in my mind was a 23-year-old boy. We don't have very many, but that was pretty horrific, because what can you say to any mother? In that situation, there's not one word of comfort we can give. We had a phone call from a doctor in Canada saying that he had an unusual cancer, with very little time left and it has always been his dream to go to England. His mother and father had agreed. The boy got here with his best friend. So two teenage boys, slightly punky-looking, walk in here and the boy looked not too bad, but we knew the medical history. We gave them a room, they went out on the town. He was here for not very long and died.

Everybody was terribly upset. No way you couldn't be. We had a beautiful little service for him here. Very tough. It was beautiful for his mum and dad, because they loved the fact that we cared for him. It was a relief to them, everything was taken care of. They were caring, thoughtful people and they were very worried about the young friend who did a great job of looking after him.

Louise

Others are remembered for other qualities:

I've got a lady aged 98. She's fighting. She has something to live for – she hasn't told me what it is yet. She's got a good relationship with me. Looking at her clinically, I don't know how she's done so well. It's end stage heart failure and there are all sorts of difficult things, but she's fighting on. She's a real sweetie. She gave me some chocolates for Easter. She has had a long life, very long.

Vicky

There's one wonderful man here who's got the whole of his face gone and he just never ceases to amaze me. His eyes are permanently bandaged up and last week with the heat, he looked awful, but he was always very chatty.

He's inspiring. The man hasn't seen for years and they have to keep changing the bandages – I think sometimes it's only due to the grace of God that people have some incredible resources to call upon.

Matthew

There was a lady who reminded me of my mum. She had dementia – she used to wander and she would come in and sit with me, she thought she worked with me. We used to sit together and chat and she called me the boss. She was gorgeous. I felt very protective of her. I was so glad when she died with us, because she should have gone to a nursing home, but she didn't. I felt that she wouldn't have been looked after and she wouldn't have been loved. She was loved here.

Carole

There was a lady who, for the first eight weeks, would come in and immediately sit down in one of our big chairs, get the newspaper, open it fully and hold it so that it hid her face. She would put it down at lunchtime and eat with the others, so we could connect with her from time to time. When I talked with staff, I would suggest this lady is coming to us under her own terms, so don't try and make her put the paper down, just connect with her every so often – hello, cup of tea, whatever. She didn't say anything to anybody, she'd have her lunch, she'd go back to the same big chair, the paper would go up again – for about eight weeks.

Then we had a meeting with patients and she sat there quietly, listening. People wanted breathing exercises – we had a patient who was a retired physiotherapist who was helping us to set them up. The 'newspaper lady' came to me in my office after the meeting and said she used to be a yoga teacher and she'd like to teach some breathing here. I said 'absolutely fabulous' – and thought here's her way in. We talked a little on how she would like to introduce it to the others. So the next time she came in, after lunch she did an experiential group on breathing. I left the room for a while and when I came back, she had one leg right over the top of her head, holding it with her hand on the other side! People were watching in complete silence, mesmerised. From there on in, she just became the most wonderful member of the community – loving and perceptive and just fabulous. It was like watching a flower blossom; she just opened up. She was with us for less than a year, and died in the hospice.

Day centre manager

Feeling valued by patients and families

Of course, nurses and others like the fact that patients and relatives greatly appreciate the care they receive. This is shown in many different ways. Some say so more or less directly:

I have had two things said by different patients at the day centre. The first one was a delightful man, the financial director of a big company. He and I had a wonderful relationship and he said to me one day, 'Max, the only good thing that ever came out about having cancer is meeting you' – and I burst out crying. Then about three months ago, one of the chaps who comes in, delightful guy, said the same thing and again, I just burst out crying. You couldn't get a better compliment than that.

Max

You get such nice compliments from families, because you've taken the strain off of them. Their biggest problem is the patient is not eating. Families sometimes have the illusion that because they are eating here, they are on the road to recovery, but it gives them maybe two or three weeks of quality life. It's wonderful to have another human being say 'you don't know how much that meant to us that mum or dad ate that food. They thoroughly enjoyed it, they talk about you coming to talk to them every day'.

Chef

It's when I go in to see a patient at home and they smile at me. People tell me that patients have said 'Vicky's coming round today, what time is Vicky coming?' – that's really nice that they actually look forward to seeing you.

Vicky

Then, there is the written word:

I've got a lot of cards and letters. I'll always keep them. I've got a little filing thing at home and sometimes if I'm putting a new one in, I'll look at the others and think God, I really helped that family a lot, I did a good job there or I wonder what happened to that family?

Louise

The letters and the postcards you get from patients' families are an eye opener. We have got a book together. It is just the nice letters from families thanking the staff, a lot of them are saying that we are 'angels' and 'special people'. It is very nice being thanked in that way. I also get thanked personally quite often.

Dan

And some get showered with gifts:

You do feel a bit embarrassed at Christmas – you open the front door and fall through it, laden down by presents. I've never been given anything really valuable. If it's money, I always ask if it's OK for me to put it into our patient amenities fund. I've been given chocolates, jumpers, books, jewellery and vast amounts of alcohol. With the chocolates and alcohol, very often I leave them on the ward and we share it out. Sometimes I take the whisky home. I don't feel it's appropriate to turn down presents. People are very hurt if you do, because there is a feeling of wanting reciprocity – people want to share with you a little bit.

Anna

I've had some really amazing gifts that have really touched me – I just think I don't deserve that at all. I've had pearls and crystal and silver – somebody knitted me a teddy bear with my name on it – just beautiful things, really thoughtful things. It's a humbling job to be in.

Michelle

Sometimes, a gift has a particular significance because of the circumstances in which it is given:

There was one particular lady who was in the last stages. I came in one day and she said 'I've been out to the shops and I've got something for you that you need, the very thing'. She was Roman Catholic (and I am not) and she gave me this little box with a rosary. I've still got it. There was something about the fact that she said 'and I've been out to the shops especially for it' – she couldn't move out of her bed.

Chaplain 3

And some gifts can be a problem:

There was a patient who donated an awful reptile to the hospice – a big, live turtle in a tank. It was disgusting, but we said 'oh, thank you very much'. The sisters bought a book on how to look after it, so we were trying our best, but it got a bit mouldy on its feet. Someone reported us to the RSPCA and a guy came and said 'I hear you are being very cruel to this reptile' – and the sister was running round 'no, no – I have got this book and we have measured the cage'. It was like a comedy show. In the end, they didn't take it away, but one of the nursing sisters wanted it and, thank God, it went.

Diana

Working with other staff

Another reward is the pleasure of working with other people at the hospice, each valuing the input of the others:

We all work fantastically well together. People can get very precious in some places about their own department, but that doesn't happen here. And it's not hierarchical. If any of us felt that the manager was out of order in any way, we wouldn't hesitate to go and talk to him – and he would listen.

Andrea

We're good as a team. Sometimes, I ask the experienced nurses their view on a medical situation, 'you've worked with this patient much more, what do you think?' And they know much more about the relatives, because they spend more time with them. We can still be ourselves, we can joke – we can be friends and colleagues at the same time.

Doctor 2

We all fit with each other. I couldn't do my job without the nurses and they would find it difficult if I didn't do mine. We're very fortunate here. We do all value and understand each other's worth – without each other, we can't work. We're all cogs within one big wheel.

Head nurse

And feeling valued in turn:

I feel valued by staff. They show it in lots of little ways. They always say 'thank you for a nice shift' at the end of a shift, which goes a long way. Every time, they thank me or 'thanks girls, you worked really hard today' – always we get a thank you. They also bring in cakes, little goodies to show that they appreciate us. And we appreciate them, too.

Healthcare assistant 2

I don't think anybody goes round putting bunches of flowers out for me, but I feel an equal member of the healthcare team. Everybody has their role. I don't feel in any way devalued by being a volunteer.

Volunteer 2

There is a sense of give and take, looking out for each other's needs:

On previous jobs, I didn't want to go to work, I forced myself to get up in the morning. There was no support, no one to help you. If I had a problem with a client, it was pretty much 'shut up and put up with it' – no back-up, nothing. Here, I've got every bit of support I could possibly need. Even the doctors will come and ask 'are you OK?'

Megan

We all bounce off each other. You need to, because there are days when you are not feeling 100% and the others carry you. If I think one of the other staff is not having a very good day, I will go out of my way to do things. It is a bit of an unspoken thing, but you just do it.

Fiona

We get two or three days with relatives who may be difficult and you know you're going to have to look after them again and again. So it helps by just sharing with your peers, talking it over. Or asking them to change around, 'can you have those patients today, because I really need a break' – we do that for each other.

Eileen

A sense of fun

It is commonly said that people need a sense of humour to work in a hospice and it is clear that staff do have a lot of fun. This is partly to help them to cope with their experiences and the nature of the work that they do:

We had a week where we had something like eight deaths. That was absolutely mental. We just had to laugh about it. There's a lot of black humour. You have to have that, because if you seriously thought about the fact that we have eight people who we've lost in one week, we'd be 'oh, my God'.

Rebecca

There's a lot of teasing that goes on – teasing is very much a part of intimacy here. Palliative care can involve a lot of physical involvement and intimacy, and very often under humiliating and embarrassing situations for patients and staff. There's also a lot of humour in the course of conversations. I think a lot of it comes from the intimacy that people feel around each other, amongst both staff and patients.

Maggie

But a sense of fun is also directed to the patients, making their time in the hospice easier:

We'll have a joke with patients, mess around with them. We don't just go 'oh, dear', which is what all their relatives and friends do, because no one else knows what to say to them. We take the mickey all the time, but obviously only once you've got an idea of how a person will respond. Generally, it will be with the older men, 'you're only in here because you like women in uniform' and they'll say 'oh, you know!' And that's why they like being here, because it takes their mind off the fact that they're sitting here waiting to die.

Rebecca

There are people who I got on really well with, who perhaps had the same sense of humour. A prime example is a lovely woman, when I was working on nights, for whatever reason we got on really well. She wanted to get out of the bed and go to the toilet and she had slippers that wrap round with

Velcro and I put them on the wrong feet. She said 'next time, can you put them on the right feet' – so I got labels and I put 'left' and 'right' on them. Quite often, even if she didn't want anything, I'd go in and have a chat with her.

Helen

Sometimes, it is more a matter of getting a smile:

I always aim to leave a patient and family with a smile on their face. You can almost always get a smile, even if they're in the worst pain. You just make some silly remark about something you've picked up during your conversation with them and you can generate a little smile. If I walked around this ward, I guarantee I could go into every room and come out having had at least a smile. That helps me as much as them – it makes it easier to walk away, compared to walking away when someone is wallowing in grief. You can't do that – you have to turn it around.

William

And sometimes the humour is wholly unexpected:

You do need a sense of humour in this job. There was a lady whose husband used to come in and visit her every day and 'yes dear, no dear' and sit with her and all the rest of it. After he left one day, she said to me 'I haven't been able to stand him for the last 20 years – I wish he had left me years ago'. And then she added 'but how can I hurt him now?' She died a week or so after.

Fiona

We do what our patients want. For example, we had a young guy who died and he had two young daughters. They'd drawn a picture for daddy to go in his coffin and they'd given a pint of lager and cigarettes as well, because that's what they wanted in the coffin – you can't help but go 'ahhh' at that.

Laura

If you have no sense of humour, you've no sense of tragedy. Because in the most tragic situations, there can be something really quite funny. Or touching and you can only smile. I remember a man, his mother had been dead three days and he came in with a cardigan and her handbag 'because she feels the cold'. Now I know what he was thinking, 'oh, she felt the cold terribly' and then he gives me a little handbag and he wants her buried with it. It's very touching and very sad, but it's also very human. You need to smile and see the funny side.

Louise

PART IV

REFLECTIONS ON WORKING IN A HOSPICE

CHAPTER 11

Working in a hospice

Given the rewards that staff obtain from working in a hospice, it is likely that others might be interested in joining them. This chapter explores some practical aspects of such work.

Qualities needed

In the light of the complexity of hospice work, what qualities are needed to take it on? Key qualities seem to be having empathy and good listening skills:

> You need to be a good listener. You need to be able to encourage people, give them support. Encouragement in the sense of, if they ask you whether they should have a particular treatment, you help them to make the decision they want.
>
> *Vicky*

> It's not just doing things to a patient – it's actually including them. Nurses 'do to' patients a lot more in hospitals. The patients are nursed, but they're not always included in the care, because there's no time for that. Here, it is patient led, you include patients in everything you do. Asking them what they want and informing them what you're doing to them and that kind of thing. And you don't leave any stone unturned. You make sure they have every bit of information they need.
>
> *Michelle*

> When I had my first nursing interview, they asked me what would make me a good nurse and I said 'I'm interested in people. Some would call it nosy, I would call it interested'. I love to know about people's lives. We had a young lady a while ago who was the same age as me and we talked about the first time we got drunk – she died a few days later, but we'd had such a laugh just talking about that. Another lady it was about the different things her children had done in doctor's surgeries that were extremely embarrassing. It's just empathy. You need to like people. You need to want to do things for people.
>
> *Nina*

Patience is important:

> You need patience. Some patients may have cognition problems, mobility problems or difficulty with dressing, so you need patience and a willingness

to try not to take over, to encourage them to do what they can for themselves – to empower them with their own self-esteem. It's very important that the individual is given as much opportunity to be in control of their life as possible, because there is so much that they don't have a choice in or any control over. They need to maintain their own integrity and self-respect.

You're never going to make somebody better. You can't kid yourself about that. At best, you'll help somebody feel better about themselves. And perhaps ease them a little, make them feel a little bit more special for five or ten minutes – all day, if you're lucky.

Alice

You have to be somebody with a lot of patience, who wouldn't hurry someone, who could spend time with a patient or relative. And kind – if you weren't kind, you shouldn't be here.

Fiona

It is also essential to be tough:

You need to be quite well balanced and have the ability to go out that door – there's a big world out there – and get on with your life. People can come with a very do-good attitude. I can remember one girl, a long time ago – every time a patient died, she cried. She had to be counselled, made a cup of tea. To do that, working in a place like this, is no good. You're here to work.

Louise

You have to be quite tough. You have to be assertive, have good resources in terms of your own personal support outside. Some people are just more vulnerable and need more support. You have to be able to cope with the idea of death and dying.

Anna

A sense of humour can be helpful:

You definitely need a sense of humour. Sometimes when we get together, there is lots of laughter and patients and families have commented on that. We have had a couple of families who have sort of tutted 'all of you are laughing down there – don't you know somebody is ill?' But patients say 'it is lovely to hear laughter'. They don't want you going into them with a long face, looking miserable as sin. I would hate somebody to come to me, if I was ill, with all the worries of the day.

Fiona

You need a sense of humour. It's a cliché but it's very true, there is nothing like a palliative care nurse's sense of humour. Because of what you're seeing all day, if you're not able to chill out and joke, you're just going to take it all home with you and it's just going to build up and up – and you will just explode.

Jessica

But a wide range of other qualities are also noted:

You need imagination – to imagine somebody who's just been diagnosed. By the time people get to us, they've been through the awful day where they went with a mild headache to a doctor who had alarm bells ringing, somebody had to sit them down and say 'listen, this is what you've got and you've got about three months to live'. They've been through all that by the time they get here.

Louise

You need a sense of creativity. Not in the normal sense of the word, but thinking in context – what influences the state things are in and what difference a change might make. Looking at all sorts of different ways of solving a problem. Wanting to explore, to experiment, feeling empowered to try something and see what can happen. People working outside of parameters, opening up to possibilities.

Maggie

People need to be comfortable around anything. Some patients have got horrible tumours growing out of them and some people can't manage that well – patients pick that up. You need the ability to really be open with patients about the things that they are ashamed of, things that make them embarrassed.

Michelle

You need to be realistic. To appreciate that not everybody has a good death, not everybody dies nicely or quietly and there can be some emotional drawbacks. A person needs to know themselves, to make sure there's no baggage. We do look after our own, but you need to make sure there's no other issues that can't be resolved.

Nina

You need to be optimistic, rather than gloomy. To be able to walk away and come in the next day smiling again. You're not doing anyone any good by taking their grief on board. I say to volunteers, 'why are you grieving for somebody you didn't really know?' For a few of them, that's something of a shock, because it sounds quite tough, but patients are very vulnerable and we need to know why they're getting so upset.

Volunteer coordinator

Some of these characteristics are raised when nurses and others talk about themselves:

> I'm quite understanding. Somebody said to me the other day I was very humane. I hope they didn't mean that I put people out of their misery! I also like to have a laugh and a joke with the patients, unless I can see they're not happy with that and then I'd leave it.
>
> *Laura*

> I am a very strong willed person. My parents taught me that you will meet people in this world who might be richer than you, they might be more powerful than you, but they are no better than you. That has stuck in my mind all my life. And I am a great believer in dealing with the hand you have been dealt. Bad things will happen to you, but what can you salvage from it? So when people have a crisis, I am the person that says 'right, how can we solve it?'
>
> *Andrew*

> I have a lot of common sense. I do think that's been quite a strength here, just to have common sense enough to look at things and think, well, actually why are we doing it this way? I'm a 'people person'. I've always managed people, but I'm very much hands-on – if the girls need help washing up, I'll help.
>
> *Andrea*

> I've got a very good sense of humour – that gets me out of a lot of things. And an ability to laugh at myself. I'm a practical joker, but I always know it's my turn next and it has been several times. They say I'm strict but I'm fair – and that's OK by me. I've learned through the years to be as fair as possible.
>
> *Nina*

There is a view that it is a better job for older people, with some experience of life:

> Palliative care is something that you should come into after doing other things. All of us have had experience in medical and surgical, renal dialysis, things associated with cancer. You need to have done that, then come into palliative care. If you have a man with prostate cancer, it's a very personal thing with the impotence and everything, how can a young staff nurse understand how that affects a man psychologically? I think palliative care nurses should be a little bit older.
>
> *Helen*

> It's not everybody's cup of tea. You've got to be understanding, patient, kind. It helps to have had a few life experiences yourself – perhaps to be

over 40. This is not the right place for youngsters. There's too much death and they wouldn't have the understanding of it. You have your own issues going on. I don't think I could have worked here when I was young.

Megan

I worry about younger doctors coming into it at the front end of their career. I don't think I could have done this right from day one. It's a specialty that's suited to people who have spent a good period of time doing either general medicine or one of the other specialties. People at a mature point in their lives, with a bit more world experience.

Consultant

There are differing views on the value of people having experienced a death in their personal life. It is often argued that people are too vulnerable after a family bereavement and are less able to help others:

Nurses who have lost somebody can identify too much with the relatives and get over-involved. They may be satisfying their own needs, rather than those of the patient. There's a very fine line between empathising and taking over – doing what you feel you need to do, rather than what's right. The most important quality is the ability to be reflective, to actually question yourself and your own motives.

Jessica

If somebody is recently bereaved, they might need to work through their own bereavement process first. It's usually a year or two after a close bereavement before you should work here. We're human 'doings' – and then human 'beings' – when we have something to face, we sometimes face it by working. And although it might be wonderful to work through a bereavement, it might not be appropriate to be with people nearing the end of their life. You might be bringing your own emotion and putting it onto them.

Alice

But some argue that such a bereavement helped them to understand others' needs:

My mother and father died while I was working here and it made me understand how people feel when they have lost someone. You don't really understand until it has happened to you. It was hard, because I kept coming back here.

Dan

My aunt had cancer and was in a hospice. You always think this isn't going to happen to me. I devoted my life to this, so I should be rewarded with it not happening to anyone I love. I did have counselling afterwards, because I didn't want it to affect my job. But it's made me a far better nurse – I totally understand what relatives are going through because I've gone through it myself.

Rebecca

Those who have been involved in staff selection reflect on these issues from their personal experience of trying to choose people:

I'm a great one for the 'feel' of a person. I nurse with my gut and I interview with my gut as well. I sit there and think, if I was a patient, would I want you at my bedside? Does she make me feel cared about? Does she make me feel safe? The clinical stuff I can teach, but that aura around you of 'trust me, I'm going to do my best for you' – you've either got that or you haven't. I would want to hear something about giving good quality care and the words 'dignity', 'peaceful' and 'pain free'.

Jessica

Doctors need to have a passion for palliative care. During an interview, you find out where they're coming from, where they're going to. You ask questions about people who are dying, what would they do, how would they cope in this situation, what about family. You don't always get it right, but somebody who has a passion you can't miss.

Doctor 2

And they are aware of certain common pitfalls:

Some people want to work in a hospice for the wrong reasons. One I had recently was 'I couldn't really look after my dad when he was dying and I feel I failed him – I think I should help somebody else now'. That's not a good reason, because there's lots of issues there that that person hasn't addressed. The thing you need most is to want to give really good, basic nursing care.

Nina

One of the interview questions is 'what would you do if a patient said to you they were in pain?' We've had a couple of girls who have said 'we would sit down and pray for the patient'. That is rubbish, they don't need praying – they need pain relief.

Laura

We ask them questions about how they would feel if they saw people with facial disfigurement and things like that, because we don't want people who are weak stomached. We had one woman and she didn't have an eye socket, she used to put her hands up and bring her finger out of her eye.

She was comfortable doing that – it was not for me to tell her not to. You can't just walk in and say 'I want to do good deeds'.

Andrew

Training

Much training is, of course, available. Some find that some aspects of this are very helpful in enabling them to cope:

They're very hot on the training here, so it's already organised in your start package. I've done moving and handling, first aid, manual handling, fire training. You have to renew them – they only last for six months or a year and then you do them again. Some could be a couple of hours, some could be all day. I found the counselling course extremely helpful – if a patient asks you a question, how to answer it. When I first started, I'd say I'll go get somebody, but now I can often deal with it myself.

Megan

I did a two-day course on facing up to your fears about dying. They take you to a time of your earliest memory of death – how you felt about it, what you would have wanted from it. That was across the board – people who had been evacuated in the war and somebody who lost their husband suddenly, when he'd had a heart attack in the garage. That helped me an awful lot.

Laura

I attended a one-year crash course in social work and counselling and I spent three months in a local children's department working as a social worker. With the best will in the world, priests may not always have the skills to help people, for example counselling. I found the course invaluable. You not only look at the presenting symptoms, but try to look underneath. This is vital for most priests nowadays.

Chaplain 1

The occasional course may be seen as unimpressive:

When I started in this field, I went to do a natural death centre course on coping with death. It was utterly silly. You had to walk round with your eyes closed, as though that had anything to do with being dead! Then you had to get into pairs and one person had to pretend to be Death and speak to the other. So this girl said to me 'I am Death and you're floating away on a cloud and your family are around the bed and they're holding your hand.' When it was my turn, I said 'I am Death and you've gone out across the road and you've just been killed and your children are at home and they don't know you've popped out to the shops' and she cried her eyes out. I thought you ought to think about your own death when you're working with people who have got to face theirs.

Anna

A lot of training will be in-house from experienced staff:

One of my jobs is to be a kind of practice facilitator, particularly with new staff. I teach them how to carry out certain procedures, the way that we do it. Our standards are quite high and, although it may be acceptable somewhere else, it may not be acceptable here. We will make sure that we show them the way we want things done.

Head nurse

We've run training sessions with some of our administrative staff, because they may see a patient or get the odd phone call. We've done some really good training on boundaries. They've all got kids and the kids mess them around at times and we say 'well, put some boundaries in place – this is what you'll accept and this is what you won't accept'. It's almost like a garden fence – this is my garden fence, you're allowed up to that point and you can come in if I invite you, but otherwise you stay there.

Counsellor 2

But it is often felt that there is no substitute for experience:

However much you do courses, it doesn't really prepare you to work with death and dying – or even get an understanding of how much people want to talk or not talk. You need to learn the signals. I'd worked in a lot of different settings, so I had a good grounding, but to actually be thrown in at in the deep end was very frightening. The hospice had a fantastic nursing team and they taught me so much – the old nurses knew their stuff.

Andrea

A lot of this job is learning from the people who you work with. Everybody who works in this place has got something to give. Some might be better listeners, some might be excellent at wound care, but the fact that they work here makes them want to do something more than an average job. It's watching experienced nurses, for instance you don't bang the door open and just walk in and say 'morning!' That's not appropriate when somebody is feeling really rough. So it is just observing and learning.

Fiona

Telling people what you do

One of the odder difficulties of working in a hospice is telling other people what you do. This is mainly because people are uncomfortable around the idea of dying and cannot imagine why anyone would choose to work with it on a daily basis:

There's one way to end a conversation and that's to tell someone what I do for a living. People don't want to talk about death at all. If the conversation does go on, they might say their mother has cancer and all of a sudden I find myself talking to a complete stranger about things that are really quite intimate.

Rebecca

The other day I met a lady who asked how I could work here. I said it's because I like it, it's what I want to do. A lot of people are afraid of death and dying. I've had a few people ask why I don't work in a hospital. It's really hard to explain why.

Grace

Friends ask me – one asked me this morning – 'how do you do the job you do?' I said 'that's a very good question – I have never been able to answer it. It is just something that you cope with, your mind tells you, you can cope'. Even my own GP has asked me the same question 'how do you do that job?' I said I don't know. Same question, same answer.

Dan

There tend to be two common responses:

I don't tell anybody what I do. Because they either say 'oh isn't it depressing – how can you do that?' or 'I just so admire you'. I get really sick of hearing it, so I just tell people I'm a nurse. Otherwise you just get into this conversation about death and dying. I just want my friends to know me as me, not as a nurse caring for people who are dying.

Laura

You get two attitudes. Some people think 'oh my God, I couldn't do that – you're so wonderful'. Others think 'I don't want to know about that – thanks, but no thanks'. Or they ask me 'isn't that terribly depressing? Don't you feel terribly depressed all the time?'

Anna

When people say 'what do you do?' I always hesitate because, when I tell them, there is a sort of shock, horror – and then people say 'oh, you must be an amazing person'. And I say 'no, just an ordinary person'.

Claire

CHAPTER 12

Reflections on living and dying

Those who work daily with people who are dying almost inevitably ponder a number of issues concerning both dying and living. This chapter explores some reflections arising from such work.

A good death

Working with dying people means a concern with providing what is often called 'a good death'. There are differing views about what this entails, but it is commonly seen as being peaceful and pain-free:

> In a good death, it's peaceful, they're not in pain, they're ready. Some people actually say 'I'm ready now, everything's done, I don't feel uncomfortable' and it's a peaceful experience. It's always traumatic, but if it's as good as you could possibly do it, then that's a good death.
>
> *Catherine*

> A good death is both physical and emotional. If people are physically in pain, often they are emotionally in pain or turmoil. So the good scenario would be that you resolve that and then they start to relax and are not in pain. That does happen. They come in here and they feel safe – they are able to let go and get their life sorted at the end.
>
> *Claire*

It is also important that relatives perceive it as peaceful:

> Sometimes it seems like a good death to us, because we are used to seeing people die in different ways, but a relative who's never seen anybody die may feel it wasn't. It's better when I know that the patient has died peacefully and the relatives see it that way.
>
> *Grace*

> For me, a good death is no distress, no pain and they're dignified. But it's not just for the patient, a lot of it is for the relative, because this is what's going to stay with them. From their viewpoint, a death may appear horrendous, because this is the first death they've seen. The patient may have had a very slight rattle and to the relative that could be the most horrendous

thing they've ever heard – they could walk away feeling like that person has suffered. So a 'good death' is a case of personal perceptions.

Jessica

But not everyone sees this as a straightforward issue:

I think the idea of a good death is very problematic. You have to plan for the worst and hope for the best. You don't always have control over everything. It's a bit like making a birth plan – it isn't necessarily going to go the way you want. I never made a birth plan, but some have and then they have emergency caesareans. It's a little bit like that with death.

Anna

Woody Allen said about death 'I have absolutely no fear at all about dying – it's just that I don't want to be there when it happens'. I think that's good. No matter how much training you have and how much you talk about coming to terms with it, the truth is who the hell wants to come to terms with that?

Louise

Some contrast these views with other experiences:

Some deaths are horrendous. On my last job, a palliative care ward in a hospital, we had a young girl with a determined mother who knew far better than we did. The girl was very poorly, but she wanted to get onto a chair. We were very busy with other patients and said we would come shortly to help her move. But the mother tried to move her daughter herself and the girl ended up falling on the floor and was killed from the impact. There was blood, faeces and vomit everywhere. We heard a scream, went in, and got the mother out. We had to get all the furniture out, hoist the dead girl onto the bed, clean the entire area – all as fast as possible, because the mother was banging the door down wanting to come in. She swore horrendously and told us it was our fault. Later, I went home and burst into tears.

Rebecca

I've worked in casualty and in intensive care where there's been traumatic death – where relatives are not expecting it, they haven't spoken to that person, they haven't told them that they love them – that's horrendous and people are left unsatisfied.

Catherine

Choosing the timing of death

It is commonly said that people are able to select the timing of their death. Many hospice staff agree with this. It is said that some people decide the time is coming and begin to let themselves go:

> I think people do choose when they die. They lose that sparkle, they lose something within their eyes – that says to me 'I haven't got long'. If they want to die, they will die. One lady constantly kept saying 'I don't know why I wake up in the morning – I don't want to be here' and a week later she died. It's just a kind of feeling. There is something that says they're dying.
>
> *Vicky*

> I believe people do make the choice to move toward death, based on conversations I've had. One HIV client who had been unwell for a while came in one day to the office and said 'I can't do this anymore'. He died about a week later. Another example is a lady who said 'I have had a wonderful life'. I remember paying attention to the past tense although she still looked well. And a few days later she was dying. Maybe people have an awareness that they're experiencing a last burst of energy, or an awareness of things changing which are only tangible to them.
>
> *Day centre manager*

Many speak of people waiting for a particular event:

> I used to think that was an old wives tale. People would say 'she waited till her daughter's birthday' and you think 'oh, come on!' But you see it a lot. Maybe they wait to hear someone's voice, they wait for a date. It has happened so often that I can't believe that it's just a coincidence – the subconscious is obviously going on.
>
> *Fiona*

> There have been a few cases where patients have had relatives coming from far away. We had family coming from Australia, and the patient had deteriorated and deteriorated and I thought he wouldn't last till the family came. But surprisingly he did and a couple of hours later he died. So maybe that's what he was waiting for.
>
> *Julia*

> I've known many patients who say 'I just want to see Christmas', 'I want to see the grandchildren', 'I want to see if she has a boy or a girl', 'I want to see Easter out'. If the will is there and if they're waiting to see someone, it is often the case.
>
> *Alice*

This is so common that when a patient has remained alive beyond what was expected, staff begin to question whether he or she is waiting for something:

We often say that when someone's not going, there's a reason. And then we will go through everything – has every family member been? Has there been a feud? Is something going on? I think there's an added peace for the person going and for the person left behind.

Michelle

There are times when you think 'my goodness, that patient certainly physically, medically should be dead', but they will carry on for a week or two, to see their son or to hang on for Christmas or anniversaries – and then deteriorate very quickly. There tend to be more deaths after holidays, such as Christmas.

Diana

There are also patients who simply want to get their house in order:

We have a lady at the moment – she was a professional person and she's lived quite an independent life. She's always made arrangements and now at the end of her life, she has arranged her funeral. She has taken great pains to make sure her will is written and she's been hanging on, just to make these last arrangements. Every day, she's a little bit weaker, but she's done a bit more. She's had a solicitor in to visit this week, she's had a priest in and now she's not able to talk. She's allowed us to wash her and all of those things, which last week she would never have done.

From the moment she came in, she's just had such peace, 'I am able enough to do the things I want to do – all I want now is to prepare a few things and I'm ready to die'. It's just lovely to hear someone say 'I'm at peace' and really mean it – very sincerely mean it.

Eileen

In addition to waiting for a particular event, people are also thought to choose the moment in the day, perhaps when their family are present:

We always make it very clear to relatives that they must keep talking to the patient – they know you're here, tell them who's in the room, tell them everything you've always wanted to tell them and tell them they can go. I think it's only natural that we walk in the room and we say 'you're all right now, everything's safe, everyone is here you love – just relax, just go'.

Rebecca

One woman was so frightened that she would not be there when her mum passed away that she was here for weeks. And when it happened, her mum had been unconscious for days, but she actually felt that she brightened up, looked up and reached out for her. Quite amazing.

Catherine

But it also seems to work in the opposite way – that patients die in the few moments when family members are out of the room:

> There have been cases where the patient wants to die on their own. I remember one family where all the sisters, mother and mother-in-law made sure there was always someone in the room. The patient had deteriorated and we knew that it was going to be at any time, but something happened that they all needed to go out – perhaps to move the car – and he died whilst they were all outside of the room. It was just the five minutes that they were away. He had just gone. Maybe he didn't feel they could cope to be in the room. I don't know. People try to protect their loved ones.
>
> *Julia*

> There was one young woman, whose husband was anxious all the time and she was nearing the end. She was a very gentle lady – she asked him to go downstairs and make her a cup of tea. And while he was out of the room, she died. It was almost as if she had wanted him to go to let her just go. And it is an odd thing to ask somebody if you know you are dying 'could you go and make me a cup of tea?' A very kind thing to do. I think he understood that was her way of doing things.
>
> *Carole*

Occasionally, this is the source of some anger from relatives:

> Relatives could be in here for days and then just miss that moment. It's awful when they do. There is often anger. They write to me – they expect, in a hospice, for you to be able to predict it, that you know the exact time and date. It's not an exact science, unfortunately. It is a very difficult one – we always try to monitor people closely to make sure that we give relatives enough notice so that they can be there, but sadly, that doesn't always happen.
>
> *Head of hospice 1*

What happens after death?

It seems very natural for people who work with those who are dying to reflect, as people tend to do from time to time, on what happens after death. There are those who stress that they do not know any better than anyone else:

> I wish I knew! I haven't actually had a single patient asking that, but I don't know what I would answer. Sometimes you can see from the facial expressions that they are comfortable. But I wouldn't know what happens after we've died.
>
> *Julia*

I haven't a clue what happens when we die. I'd love to believe we all meet up with our old friends and have a great time, but I'm not sure I can buy that one, eternal life. There's a part of me that more and more thinks there's maybe some kind of spiritual thing that goes on afterwards, but it's not something I dwell on.

Louise

Some believe in the existence of an afterlife of one kind or another:

None of us knows exactly, but as a Christian I believe that I'm safe in the hands of God. Patients don't ask me about this and I wouldn't see it as my role to raise the subject. I'm listening for what's said and unsaid. I might ask if I felt somebody was worried or frightened and that might lead on to the subject, but I certainly wouldn't offer it. Other chaplains might feel that was a stronger part of what they were about.

Chaplain 3

I feel that people go somewhere else – to meet their God, their Maker, their Allah or whatever. It's not that common for people to talk about these things. Some people just feel that their mother or their sister will be there and that's good enough, they don't feel that they're going to be at a loss, there will be someone there for them.

Eileen

And some feel it would be nice to do so:

I do envy people who have a strong faith, who actually have somewhere they believe they're going. If you've got a terminal disease and you think this is what God's given me, you'll put up with this, because when I die, God is going to reward me. It must be wonderful to believe that. They seem to die more peacefully.

Helen

I think it's nice to have something to believe in – whether you're a Buddhist, Catholic or whatever. We had a lady once who was a Spiritualist – she painted a picture of where she was going to go after she died. It was a little stream with a lovely blossomed tree hanging over and it was a brilliant sunny day – it was just her leaning up against the tree and that's where she wanted to be. And I thought, 'that's lovely'.

Laura

Others are quite certain that there is nothing more after life:

I don't believe there's an afterlife. When you're dead, you're dead. We go into the earth and disintegrate. If there was a heaven, it would have to be a jolly big place. As a Jewish man, our holy days are New Year and ten days later it's the Day of Atonement. It used to be said that God looks at your records on the New Year and, between then and the Day of Atonement, decides who's going to live and who's going to die, who's going to be rich, who's going to be poor, who's going to suffer and so on. As a child, I used to sit in the synagogue with my father and brothers and I had this vision of this long-haired, white-bearded person in a big white robe with a piece of paper in his hand, ticking off, 'die', 'live', 'rich', 'poor'.

Max

Some stress that they are much more interested in what happens in this world:

I believe when people pass on, they can still be influential in some way or another, that something about them being in this world made a difference and that difference continues. What happens here, what makes a difference here, is what's more important to me.

Maggie

I feel the only immortality we have is how we're remembered by our family and friends. One of the most important things to me is that I would matter to my children. I was taking a walk with one of my daughters last summer and she said 'I've decided if you could live to be 103, I'd be 73, then it would be OK if you died'. I said I couldn't possibly arrange to live to be 103! But it's that sense that they would remember me as somebody who had been important in their lives.

Anna

Some fear that palliative care is too much wrapped up in religion:

For some staff, a belief in the afterlife is why they do it – they have a more spiritual approach to death. I'm always uncomfortable with it impinging on what we're doing and I worry when people throw it in. That can turn a lot of people off. Some patients have a preconception that they're going to have religion thrown down their throats in a hospice – and if they've never been a believer, they don't want any of that. That doesn't happen here, but I have worked in some hospices where a strong religious belief was known to be there.

William

There is also an argument for a need for much better preparation for death:

Life is a rehearsal for death and none of us can avoid it. We have midwives for people coming in, but we don't prepare for death in any way. We don't talk about it, we don't know how to handle it and we do not accept death. We shut people away when they're dying – it's a very hidden thing from our young. You might see it on the TV, but it's not real.

Within my own family, it's never been an issue. My mum will say to me 'right, I'm clearing my house out, so you won't have to when I die – do you want this?' And it's just lovely. Very practical. I haven't been brought up with a fear of death or dying.

Alice

A sense of mortality

Working in a hospice clearly makes people very aware of their own death at some point. This has a number of specific effects. Some think about what sort of death they would prefer:

I was talking to a nurse whose father had just died of a heart attack and she was saying there was nobody with him. I said, 'at least he went there and then – just look at people who have labouring deaths, having to be turned every two hours, incontinent and so forth – which death would you rather have?' I'd rather go oomph.

Helen

We all think about our own mortality. You see what the patients are like and we think, 'if I ever get cancer, just shoot me'. I want to die quietly, calmly and free from pain – in a hospice.

Dan

Some had thought about death long before coming to the hospice:

Death used to be referred to as 'pushing up daisies'. I used to imagine myself lying under the ground in this beautiful warm, brown soil, pushing flowers up and I thought that would be great. I've never been frightened of death or dying. I don't want a painful death, but I've been brought up to accept the fact without it being made a horror or anything. But I don't want loose ends – I wouldn't like to think that I left debts for my children.

Alice

Death used to terrify me. Even as a little girl, if I had a bad dream or something to do with death, I used to say to myself 'no, I've got to grow up first and be a mother and a grandmother'. It did used to frighten the life out of me. I've got over it since I've come here. I was in the mortuary within two hours of starting – they said the quicker I got in there, the better it would be for me – and it worked. I've never looked back.

Megan

It also makes staff generally more aware of diseases:

If you go home and you have a sore head, you think maybe it's a brain tumour. If I have a pain in my back, I might think maybe I've got cancer that's spread to my bones. These thoughts don't last very long, but if I weren't working in a hospice they wouldn't really cross my mind.

Charlotte

Having worked here, I've decided there's nothing I want to die of! There's no disease I'm prepared to have, so I'll have to face that when I get to it. It would be awfully hard if you were a hypochondriac and working in a hospice! It does make me more aware of mortality, but I don't worry about dying particularly. Obviously, I hope it will be quite a long way off, as there are quite a lot of things I'd like to do before I die.

Anna

And sometimes other dangers:

There isn't a day goes by without me thinking at some point, here I am and I could not be here in the next second. I feel particularly mortal on the street. I could be at traffic lights and think I'm going to wait, rather than run for it, because if I don't, this could be the day when some asshole in their car runs the red light. I find it really interesting to feel mortal, to feel that sense of taking care.

Maggie

For some, it has a practical effect, for instance giving attention to wills:

I'm pushing my parents all the time to write a will. We have people who are supposed to sign their will in the morning and they just die and it's too late. I don't know what happens then – we don't get involved in any of that. I knew a woman in my previous job who had a horrendous ex-husband and she'd met a new man and it was fantastic, and then she became extremely ill. The new man brought the will in for her to adjust, but she died, having left everything to the ex-husband. It was very distressing.

Rebecca

My husband and I talked about our wills last night. I just said if one of us was to die tomorrow, I'd want that the pair of us had expressed how we'd sort out our finances. We don't want to see families at war. I thought about this because I've been called out to sign wills.

Catherine

And some think about the need to prepare others for the possibility:

I do try to prepare my family. My daughter doesn't really want to know, my son's much more realistic. I'm not saying he'd find it any easier, but my daughter is really fearful about anything happening to me. You see so many daughters who live in their mother's pocket all the time – they go shopping together, they do everything together – and when mum dies, they've got nothing. I make sure my daughter isn't in that situation. I see her once a week and I talk to her a lot on the phone. We are a very close family, but they're all independent and they're all doing their thing.

Andrea

Learning what is important

Working in a hospice seems to bring many insights to people. A common one is the need to do the things you most want to do, because of the brevity of life:

Being around death teaches you to enjoy yourself. There was a very old doctor when I first came here. He was a very wise medical guy and a very interesting man, rather grand and flamboyant. He used to come and have a chat and he said something to me that I never, ever forgot. He said 'keep away from the surgeons, my dear' – he was a surgeon – 'keep away from the surgeons and enjoy yourself. We're only here for the weekend'. I never forgot that.

Louise

Working with dying people makes me think about living a bit more. I want to cram it all in, I want to do all the holidays. There has never been anybody who said 'I should have worked more hours, done my housework, gone out and earned loads of money'. One gentleman said to me 'if you have got friends, you have got everything. If you have got family, you have got everything. If you have got debt, don't worry about it, they can't hang you for it'. I have had lots of really good advice down the years.

Fiona

Some note that this is easier said than done:

I wish I could live via my own dictates of living each day to the full and not worrying about whatever, but of course nobody ever does. It's quite hard to do that in the real world – the ordinary worries of everyday life overtake you. But you never know if you're going to fulfil your retirement plans and it is quite a good idea to do nice things when you want to do them and not put them off, because you might not ever get to do them. I wish I had a pound for every time I've met somebody who's going to do something in particular when they retire and then it all went wrong and it never happened.

Anna

The importance of relationships – and respecting other people – is recognised:

It teaches you about value of each day. There's more to life than having loads of money – it's all about time and friends and family. The best gift you can give to anybody is time. Just time to be with somebody – spending time with family and friends, you can never get that back. You actually don't know when's the last time you're going to see somebody – don't end on a bad note, don't have an argument with them, life's too short. It has changed the way that I look at things.

Catherine

I used to bear a grudge easily, but I can't be bothered now – life's too short. If you don't want to talk to me, fine, come and talk to me when you want to, but I can't be worrying about it. It's also made me appreciate my extended family a bit more. Aunts and uncles that have fallen by the wayside over the years – you realise they're not going to be there forever.

It makes you look at people a bit more. When I'm walking up the high street, I always get behind the person that's got nowhere to go and all day to get there – I still get slightly irritated, but whereas before I would tut, I now think it could be me one day. I think I'm a less judgemental person. I hope it's made me a nicer person.

Nina

Two things have struck me very strongly. One is the number of people who have said things like 'I didn't realise what it was to be alive' and then they put attention into life. The other is the fact that relationships are important. I was brought up with 'never go to bed on an argument'. And it really is quite devastating for people if they lose a loved one on bad terms. I've become aware of the importance of living fully, being aware of what you're doing and who you're with.

Alice

Family becomes particularly important:

Working in a hospice has made me realise how lucky I am – I'm a healthy person, I've got a healthy family and I can't see my end in sight. But I realise that it could change at any day, so I take each day as it comes. My husband and I go on holidays three or four times a year. Quality of life is worth everything. The house will be there when I'm dead and gone – the extension can take ten years, as long as we still have the time together.

Nina

It makes you look at your own life and your family – you see what life is about. I used to have thoughts of if I lost them, how it would be telling them how I feel about them, given that opportunity. And trying to get them to look at their lives and the importance of not just sitting around, but actively enjoying life, because it can be taken away from you just like that.

Vicky

Some feel they have learned something about coping with their own death, when their time comes:

> I've had lots of gems from people at the end of their lives. I hope that I'll take them into my journey of end of life. Somehow, there's a calm and peace about them and a graciousness. I would find the stripping of my independence quite difficult to deal with, but after this experience, I hope I will be less agitated by it.
>
> *Nicola*

> I am inspired by the patients. I'm not exactly a patient man myself and I think how on earth do some of them cope? We don't get supernatural help with these things. Our faith helps us, but we think and feel the same as everybody else. Once an actor came to talk to us and he asked, about a situation, 'what would a priest think of doing?' and I said 'the same as everybody else'. People always think that you have a kind of special channel, but you just have a larger horizon.
>
> *Chaplain 1*

And some feel it helped them to cope with the death of someone close to them:

> The most important thing I've learned is in relation to my mum. She had chronic illnesses, so for some years prior to her death, I knew it was going to come at some point. I learned to ask her what she wanted, instead of deciding everything for her. Working here showed me that what I thought was quality of life was not necessarily what she thought. It was a case of sitting down with her and asking her what she wanted at the end. She changed her mind several times, but in the end, she did want to be resuscitated, even though it was going to be hopeless. I went with that and I'm glad I did, because she felt that she had an advocate. She knew that I was the one that would stand up for her and say 'look, this is what she wants'.
>
> *Jessica*

Extending the learning from hospice care

Perhaps it is right to end on some ideas for improving palliative care beyond the hospice setting:

> Just because someone has to die in the hospital, there's no reason why they can't die just as they do in the hospice. It distresses me when I see things go wrong, because the right people are not there to look after them. So one of our main goals is training hospital doctors and nurses by example.
>
> Actually knowing when someone is dying is still the hardest thing, recognising that really there's nothing more you're going to do that's going to change the course of events. That's the biggest barrier – and that's what

I do day after day with the nurses I work with. We help them to come to the realisation that 'hey, guys, we've done all we can for this patient now – there isn't anything more and the kindest thing is to back off.' Some families can be very pushy about wanting to maintain treatment that's futile, so it's being able to recognise when it is – and convey that to families and patients. It's all communication, but you have to be very clear in your own mind that this is where you're at – and that's hard.

In some countries, palliative care is within a general hospital, with a ward for palliative care. That's a good model of how to manage terminally ill patients within a general hospital setting. It's not necessarily preferable, because the atmosphere you can provide within a hospice is often very different, but you can make a hospital ward very homely. Then, everybody else in the general hospital can see how to manage people in the terminal phase, so it's a good learning place for care of the dying.

Patients who are terminally ill can be brought from around the hospital onto the palliative care ward. If it is very close to other wards, nurses on other wards can use it as a resource if they need help or advice. I would like to see that here in Britain. We've talked about it in the local hospital and they may give us a few beds on one of the general wards to be entirely for palliative care, where we could train nurses. It would be a model of end of life care for the general hospital. Hospitals are still places where sick people come to die. Patients can't all come to a hospice, there's just not enough beds, so we need to bring hospice attitudes into the hospital. I think this will be the natural extension of hospice care.

Consultant